U0265186

军事医学英语阅读教程

主编　姜琳琳　李　佳

南开大学出版社

天　津

图书在版编目(CIP)数据

军事医学英语阅读教程 / 姜琳琳，李佳主编. 一天津:南开大学出版社，2022.1
ISBN 978-7-310-06238-6

Ⅰ.①军… Ⅱ.①姜… ②李… Ⅲ.①军事医学－英语－阅读教学－军事院校－教材 Ⅳ.①R82

中国版本图书馆 CIP 数据核字(2021)第 273376 号

军事医学英语阅读教程
JUNSHI YIXUE YINGYU YUEDU JIAOCHENG

南开大学出版社出版发行
出版人:陈　敬
地址:天津市南开区卫津路 94 号　　邮政编码:300071
营销部电话:(022)23508339　营销部传真:(022)23508542
https://nkup.nankai.edu.cn

河北文曲印刷有限公司印刷　全国各地新华书店经销
2022 年 1 月第 1 版　　2022 年 1 月第 1 次印刷
260×185 毫米　16 开本　11.5 印张　1 插页　291 千字
定价:38.00 元

如遇图书印装质量问题,请与本社营销部联系调换,电话:(022)23508339

《军事医学英语阅读教程》编写组

主　编　姜琳琳　李　佳

副主编　张武萍　鲍玉荣　石　洁　潘俊峰

编　者　陈　蓉　张雪燕　张　玲

编者的话

前言《军事医学阅读教程》

为了突出强军目标和备战打仗要求，立起军队英语教学"姓军为战"的鲜明导向，近年来我们在研究生英语教学中增加了"军事医学英语"课程，旨在通过对军事医学的前沿问题研究，切实提升学员对外军事交流能力和卫勤保障专业素养，为培养国际化高层次军事医学人才提供有力支撑。

作为军事医学院校硕博研究生"军事医学英语"课程配套教材，《军事医学英语阅读教程》共分 10 个单元，内容包括联合国军事卫勤相关政策及军事医学前沿研究文献，每个单元分为精读课文 A 篇、词汇、注释、练习和扩展等环节，可供课堂教学使用，阅读课文 B 篇、词汇、注释，可供课后学生扩展使用，此外还给学生提供课后自我学习阅读所需的网站信息等。

本教材依据专门用途英语（English for Specific Purpose，ESP）教学理论，从当前军事医学院校研究生的应用需求和语言能力分析入手，按照循序渐进的教学原则编写而成。课文内容全部选自近几年国际军事医学网站和主流期刊发表的前沿研究文献，由解放军总医院研究生院外语教研室、解放军总医院军事医学专家团队、国防大学及军事科学院军事卫勤专家选材和编写，适用于军事医学院校硕博士研究生，也适合高等院校非英语专业国防生，以及部队科研院所的官兵使用。

借此机会感谢为本书出版提供全方位支持的解放军总医院研究生院领导，感谢课文原文作者解放军总医院付小兵院士、黎檀实主任、李春宝主任等，感谢为译文术语把关的解放军军事科学院王磊主任、付征南研究员、方明研究员等。由于编者水平有限，书中难免有不足之处，敬请读者批评指正。

编写团队

2021 年 10 月于解放军总医院研究生院

Contents

Unit One Missions for World Peace

Text A
China's Armed Forces: A Key Force in UNPKOs

Over the past 30 years, China's armed forces have contributed a growing number of peacekeepers across an expanding range of deployments. From a few military observers at the outset of its involvement, China's armed forces are now sending both formed units and military professionals. Chinese military peacekeepers serve on the UN missions in engineer, medical, transport, helicopter, force protection and infantry units, and as staff officers, military observers and seconded officers. Chinese military peacekeepers have left their footprints in over 20 countries and regions including Cambodia, the Democratic Republic of the Congo (DRC), Liberia, Sudan, Lebanon, Cyprus, South Sudan, Mali and the Central African Republic. They have made a tremendous contribution to facilitating the peaceful settlement of disputes, safeguarding regional security and stability, and promoting economic and social development in host nations.

1. Ceasefire Supervision

Ceasefires are supervised to ensure that conflicting parties abide by their agreements. It was the earliest function of UN peacekeeping, and the first task undertaken by Chinese military peacekeepers. Since 1990, in addition to military observers, more military professionals have been involved in UN peacekeeping as staff officers and seconded officers. In the past three decades, China's armed forces have sent 2,064 military professionals to 25 missions and UN headquarters (UNHQ). Thirteen of them have been appointed to key positions as force commander, deputy force commander, sector commander, and deputy sector commander. In August 2020, 84 military professionals were working on missions and at UNHQ on patrols, observation, ceasefire supervision, liaison, negotiation, command and control, and operations planning.

Military observers are deployed in conflicts to gather information for decision making. Their lives are often threatened by armed conflicts. On July 25, 2006, during the Israel-Lebanon conflict, Du Zhaoyu, a young Chinese military observer deployed in south Lebanon, bravely remained at his post, fulfilled his duty, and made the ultimate sacrifice for peace. He was posthumously awarded First Class Merit by the Chinese military and the Dag Hammarskjöld Medal[1] by the UN.

2. Stabilizing the Situation

Promptly stabilizing the situation paves the way for the peace process. This is a main task of UN peacekeeping missions, and an important area to which Chinese peacekeeping troops have expanded their functions in recent years. The security situation in some mission areas is challenging, marred by frequent conflicts, terrorist attacks and violent riots. Among all peacekeeping units, it is the infantry battalions that are mainly tasked with armed patrol, separating conflicting parties, riot control, cordoning, and search. They are the backbone for UN peacekeeping and the stabilizers of security.

In January 2015, the Chinese People's Liberation Army (PLA) dispatched an infantry battalion of 700 troops to the United Nations Mission in South Sudan (UNMISS)[2], the first organic unit of its kind to operate overseas in a peacekeeping mission. Over the past five years, six rotations have been committed to UNMISS. The Chinese infantrymen worked day and night amid the rattle of gunfire and the rumble of explosions in the mission area. As of August 2020, these battalions had completed 51 long-range and 93 short-distance patrols, 314 armed escorts, and over 30,000 hours of patrols in weapons-free zones, making a significant contribution to stabilizing the local situation. In August 2018, when a large riot erupted in Juba, capital of South Sudan, the Chinese infantry battalion acted immediately on orders and quelled the violence decisively and promptly.

3. Protecting Civilians

The Protection of Civilians (POC) is an important part of the UNPKOs. It is a duty that Chinese military peacekeepers resolutely undertake. The Chinese people suffered immensely from the scourge of war in modern times, and Chinese service members know only too well the value of peace and life. In war-torn mission areas, Chinese military peacekeepers maintain peace with their sweat, youth and lives.

In July 2016, an armed conflict broke out in Juba between government and opposition forces. Heavy weapons including tanks, large-caliber artillery, and armed helicopters were employed by both sides in fierce exchange of fire, putting a large number of civilians in severe danger. The Chinese infantry battalion, together with peacekeepers from other countries, was responsible for protecting civilians in downtown Juba and over a hundred surrounding villages. Facing a raging storm of gunfire and artillery bombardment, the Chinese infantrymen risked their lives to build a defense for life and prevented the militants from approaching the POC camp, and ensured the safety of over 9,000 civilians. Corporal Li Lei and Sergeant Yang Shupeng sacrificed their lives in the action. They lived up to the solemn pledge and sacred obligation of protecting lives and safeguarding peace with bravery and sacrifice. They were posthumously conferred First Class Merit by the Chinese military and the Dag Hammarskjöld Medal by the UN.

4. Providing Force Protection

Force protection is vital to securing the personnel and assets of UN peacekeeping missions. As an important contributor to the UNPKOs, China's armed forces have been active in sending in troops to the UN missions to provide reliable force protection.

In December 2013, China's armed forces dispatched a force protection unit of 170 troops to the United Nations Multidimensional Integrated Stabilization Mission in Mali (MINUSMA)[3] to conduct guard duties and VIP protection at the Sector East Headquarters. This was the first time that China's armed forces had dispatched troops to carry out force protection duties for the UNPKOs. Mali is among the most dangerous mission areas, afflicted by frequent suicide attacks, roadside bombs and other terrorist assaults. Over the past seven years, China's armed forces have sent 1,440 troops for force protection in eight rotations to MINUSMA. The units have fulfilled their tasks effectively in the hazardous southern edge of the Sahara Desert, including over 3,900 armed patrols and armed escorts. They have earned themselves the reputation of "des troupes d'élite[4]" of Sector East. On May 31, 2016, First Sergeant Shen Liangliang was killed trying to prevent a terrorist vehicle laden with explosives from crashing into the UN camp. He was posthumously conferred First Class Merit by the Chinese military and the Dag Hammarskjöld Medal by the UN. On the occasion of the 70th anniversary of the founding of the PRC, First Sergeant Shen Liangliang was conferred the national honorary title of People's Hero.

On March 12, 2017, an intense conflict broke out in Yei, a border town in South Sudan. Seven UN civilian staff were caught in the crossfire and they were at severe risk of losing their lives. The Chinese infantry battalion immediately sent in 12 officers and soldiers to the rescue. Despite threats and dangers in their way, they outmaneuvered the militants, defeated three interception attempts, and successfully evacuated the trapped personnel. This timely and efficient operation was hailed and publicized as an exemplary model of rescue operations by UNMISS.

5. Deploying Enabling Capabilities

Force enablers such as engineer, transport, medical, and helicopter units play an irreplaceable role in the UNPKOs. Currently, the majority of Chinese peacekeeping troops perform such enabling tasks. On UN peacekeeping missions, Chinese military peacekeepers in the logistic support units have become the embodiment of China's quality, speed and standards through their skills, professionalism and dedication.

In January 2020, some terrorists attacked the Tessalit Camp in the Sector North of MINUSMA and wounded more than 20 people. The Chinese medical unit in Sector East was rushed in by air and evacuated seven injured Chad[5] peacekeepers to the Chinese medical camp. All the wounded were saved by prompt emergency treatment. In May 2020, despite the ongoing COVID-19 pandemic and a tense security situation, the Chinese engineer unit built a bridge over the Sopo River in South Sudan to the highest quality standards. This bridge created a transport route between Wau and Raga, which was highly commended by the local government and residents.

In the past 30 years, China's armed forces have contributed 111 engineer units totaling 25,768 troops to eight UN peacekeeping missions in Cambodia, the DRC, Liberia, Sudan, Lebanon, Sudan's Darfur[6], South Sudan, and Mali. These units have built and rehabilitated more than 17,000 kilometers of roads and 300 bridges, disposed of 14,000 landmines and unexploded ordnance, and performed a large number of engineering tasks including leveling ground, renovating airports, assembling prefabricated houses, and building defense works. Twenty-seven transport units totaling 5,164 troops were dispatched to the UN peacekeeping missions in Liberia and Sudan. They transported over 1.2 million tons of materials and equipment over a total distance of more than 13 million kilometers. Eighty-five medical units of 4,259 troops were sent to six UN peacekeeping missions in the DRC, Liberia, Sudan, Lebanon, South Sudan, and Mali. They have provided medical services to over 246,000 sick and wounded people. Three helicopter units totaling 420 troops were sent to Sudan's Darfur. They completed 1,951 flight hours, transported 10,410 passengers and over 480 tons of cargo in 1,602 sorties.

6. Sowing the Seeds of Hope

It is the common aspiration of all peoples throughout the world to live a better life. Far from home, Chinese military peacekeepers have made concrete efforts to bring peace and hope to war-afflicted peoples.

To actively facilitate humanitarian assistance. Over the past 30 years, China's peacekeeping troops have worked extensively and effectively with international humanitarian agencies, and have played an active role in resettling refugees and internally displaced persons (IDPs)[7], distributing food, building refugee and IDP camps, and carrying out disaster relief tasks. In April 2020, Uvira in eastern DRC was struck by a rare flood, which posed a severe threat to the lives and property of the locals. The Chinese engineer unit was assigned to disaster relief work at the most critical moment and rushed to help reinforce levees and restore damaged bridges. They have given the locals access to help and protection, and effectively ensured the safety and security of the affected population.

To participate extensively in post-conflict reconstruction. In a post-war country or region, when a peace agreement is reached, it is essential to restore livelihoods and social order in order to prevent the recurrence of conflict and achieve lasting peace and stability. Chinese peacekeeping troops have played an active role in post-conflict reconstruction of host nations. They built important infrastructure, monitored elections, trained local doctors and nurses, and promoted environmental protection. Their efforts have been acclaimed by the governments and peoples of host nations. Darfur lies on the edge of a desert with complex geology. It is one of the regions afflicted by the world's most severe water shortages. From 2007 to 2013, Chinese military engineers drilled 14 wells in the most difficult circumstances, and effectively alleviated the problem of water scarcity for the locals.

To pass on love and care. Chinese military peacekeepers are not only guardians of peace but also messengers of friendship. The Chinese medical units in the DRC ran a twinning project in SOS Children's Village[8] Bukavu to offer help. Touched by the love and care from the units, children in the village called the female members their Chinese mothers. The consistent efforts of the Chinese units over the past 17 years have won widespread praise from the locals. In UNMISS, Chinese military peacekeepers provided agricultural techniques, farming tools and vegetable seeds to local people. They were invited by local middle schools to teach lessons on Chinese culture and language, which were very popular with the students.

Over the past 30 years, China's armed forces have contributed more than 40,000 service members to 25 UN peacekeeping missions. Sixteen Chinese military peacekeepers have sacrificed their lives for the noble cause of peace. As of August 2020, 2,521 Chinese military peacekeepers were serving on eight UN peacekeeping missions and at UNHQ. Chinese service women are playing an increasingly important role in peacekeeping. More than 1,000 female peacekeepers have worked in medical support, liaison, coordination, demining, explosive ordnance disposal, patrol, observation, gender equality promotion, protecting women and children, and other fields. They demonstrated the talent and professionalism of Chinese women on their UN missions. Chinese peacekeeping troops have been commended by the UN and the international community for their contribution. They have won honor for their country and military.

(This article is excerpted from *China's Armed Forces: 30 Years of UN Peacekeeping Operations*)

Notes

1. Dag Hammarskjöld Medal： a posthumous award given by the United Nations to military personnel, police, or civilians who lose their lives while serving in a United Nations peacekeeping operation. The medal is named after Dag Hammarskjöld, the second Secretary-General of the United Nations, who died in a plane crash in what is now Zambia in September 1961. 达格·哈马舍尔德维持和平勋章

2. the United Nations Mission in South Sudan (UNMISS): a United Nations peacekeeping mission for the recently independent South Sudan, which became independent on 9 July 2011. UNMISS was established on 8 July 2011 by United Nations Security Council Resolution 1996. 联合国南苏丹特派团

3. the United Nations Multidimensional Integrated Stabilization Mission in Mali (MINUSMA): established by Security Council resolution 2100 of 25 April 2013 to support political processes in that country and carry out a number of security-related tasks. 联合国马里多层面综合稳定团，简称联马团

4. des troupes d' élite: elite troops 战区王牌

5. Chad: officially known as the Republic of Chad, is a landlocked country in north-central Africa. It has a population of 16 million, of which 1.6 million live in the capital and largest city N'djamena. 乍得共和国

6. Darfur: a region of the western Sudan. As an administrative region, Darfur is divided into five federal states: Central Darfur, East Darfur, North Darfur, South Darfur and West Darfur. Because of the War in Darfur between Sudanese government forces and the indigenous population, the region has been in a state of humanitarian emergency and genocide since 2003. 达尔富尔

7. internally displaced persons (IDPs): persons forced or obliged to flee or to leave their homes, in particular as a result of or in order to avoid the effects of armed conflict, situations of generalised violence, violations of human rights or natural or human-made disasters, and who have not crossed an internationally recognised state border 国内流离失所者

8. SOS Children's Village: independent, non-governmental, nonprofit international development organization headquartered in Innsbruck, Austria. The organization provides humanitarian and developmental assistance to children in need and protects their interests and rights around the world. Today it is active in 135 countries and territories. 国际儿童村

Words and Expressions

1. infantry: *n.* soldiers who fight on foot rather than in tanks or on horses 步兵

2. seconded: *adj.* (an employee) be transferred temporarily to another branch, etc. （某雇员）被借调的

3. abide by: to accept or act in accordance with (a rule, decision, or recommendation) 接受；遵照（规则、决定、劝告）

4. posthumously: *adv.* used to describe something that happens after a person's death but relates to something they did before they died 死后地；身后地

5. mar: *v.* to damage or spoil something good 破坏；毁坏

6. cordon: *n.* a line or ring of police officers, soldiers, etc. guarding something or stopping people from entering or leaving a place （由警察、士兵等组成的）警戒线；封锁线

7. quell: *v.* to stop something such as violent behaviour or protests 制止；平息

8. scourge: *n.* a person or thing that causes trouble or suffering 祸根；灾害

9. caliber: *n.* the diameter of a bullet or other projectile 口径

10. bombardment: *n.* a strong and continuous attack of gunfire or bombing 轰击；轰炸

11. militant: *n.* a person using, or willing to use, force or strong pressure to achieve aims, especially to achieve social or political change 好战分子

12. confer: *v.* to give somebody an award, a university degree or a particular honour or right 授予（奖项、学位、荣誉或权利）

13. outmaneuver: *v.* to outdo, defeat, or gain an advantage over by skillful or clever maneuvering 以计谋胜过；运用策略击败

14. exemplary: *adj.* providing a good example for people to copy 典范的；可作榜样的；

可作楷模的

15. renovate: *v.* to repair and paint an old building, a piece of furniture, etc. so that it is in good condition again 修复；翻新

16. levee: *n.* a low wall built at the side of a river to prevent it from flooding 防洪堤

Exercises

I. Reading Comprehension

A. Directions: Decide whether the following statements are True or False according to the text.

1. China has been sending military troops since its involvement in UN missions.

2. Safeguarding security was the earliest function of UN peacekeeping.

3. Infantrymen are the backbone for UN peacekeeping in stabilizing security.

4. The UNMISS was the first mission that China had dispatched a force protection unit for the UNPKOs.

5. Chinese troops earned the reputation of "des troups d'elite" in MINUSMA.

6. Sacrificed Chinese serviceman Shen Liangliang was awarded the national honorary title of People's Hero.

7. Chinese infantry troops are considered the embodiment of China's quality, speed and standard.

8. Chinese medical unit in Sector East rescued many locals during the COVID-19 pandemic.

9. Monitoring elections and environmental protection are part of UN peacekeeping work in post-conflict reconstruction of host nations.

10. Sixteen Chinese servicemen sacrificed their lives in UN peacekeeping missions.

B. Directions: Answer the following questions according to your understanding of the text.

1. What tasks do Chinese military peacekeepers fulfil on UN missions? And what was the first task undertaken by them?

2. To which area do Chinese peacekeeping troops expand their functions in recent years?

3. What was the first mission that a Chinese infantry battalion participated in as peacekeepers overseas?

4. Who made the ultimate sacrifice in the armed conflict in Juba in the mid of 2016?

5. Please briefly describe the exemplary model of rescue operation in South Sudan on March 12, 2017.

6. What contributions have Chinese military peacekeepers made in the logistic support units in the past 30 years?

7. What did Chinese military do to help solve water shortages for Darfur locals?

8. Why is it said Chinese service women play an increasingly important role in

peacekeeping?

II. Vocabulary

Directions: Choose the best word or expression from the list given for each blank. Use each word or expression only once and make proper changes when necessary.

confer	exemplary	second	abide by
renovate	posthumously	mar	scourge

1. Smallpox was probably the single biggest _____ to hit North America.

2. The game was _____ by the behavior of drunken fans.

3. It is parents' responsibilities to make sure their children _____ the law.

4. The officer was _____ for duty overseas.

5. He was buried with full military honors and _____ awarded a Purple Heart.

6. We had to _____ this after the lake overflowed its banks a couple of months ago and flooded the area.

7. An _____ person may well have the great charisma to affect others but does not necessarily know how to affect others.

8. The British monarch continues to _____ knighthood on those who are outstanding in their fields of endeavor.

III. Topics for Discussion

1. How do you understand the title of this text? Why are Chinese military peacekeepers considered a key force in the UNPKOs?

2. What achievements impress you most made by Chinese military peacekeepers over the past 30 years?

3. The lives of UN peacekeepers are often threatened by armed conflicts. Please discuss with your partner the heroic deeds that you have learned about from the text.

Text B
Military Medicine in China: Old Topic, New Concept

Xiaobing Fu

Military medicine is an important field in biological and medical sciences. Military medicine plays a key role in supporting and maintaining health, in preventing injuries and diseases in military staff and in enhancing the military armed forces in times of war. In the new millennium, military activities also involve other actions such as emergent public health crises, natural disasters, emerging conflicts and anti-terrorist campaigns in times of peace. Thus, military medicine is facing new challenges and requirements with the military transformation. These requirements involve medical services in natural disasters, accidents, terrorist attacks, and in epidemiological diseases. Thus, the topic is old but has a new concept in a rapidly developing society. Amid the new military activities, such as the Chinese naval forces on escort duties in the Gulf of Aden[1], international peacekeeping activities and humanitarian relief, the military medical mission will assume more responsibility in important areas.

Military surgery and internal medicine

The armed forces are affected by many elements, such as military equipment, technology, organization and human resources; however, the most important element is "people". Maintaining physical and mental health is the fundamental element of reinforcing the armed forces, rapidly recovering from injury, and of regenerating the fighting capacity. The aim of military medical research is to serve the people and to manage people-related health problems. Traditionally, injury from weapons is called "trauma" but can be associated with many serious complications and can cause systematic reactions and internal organ damage. Such damage is the central part of war injuries but has similarities with diseases in routine healthcare; sometimes such damage is called disease trauma, injury and illness, as well as injury complicated with disease. Modern war can not only create somatic trauma and associated diseases but also involve psychological trauma. Therefore, military medicine refers to traditional military field surgery or internal medicine as well as the overall health of military staff, particularly how to manage mental stress. Currently, military surgery and internal medicine research emphasize the reform of first aid skills and equipment, regenerative medicine, etc.

In March 1999, the People's Liberation Army (PLA) Military Medical Institute (MMI) established the Military Stress Research Department, which began many research projects in this area and has accomplished fruitful research. This area has become critical to military medicine, covering issues such as how to consult for mental health and how to establish psychological-stress standard measurements and management guidelines.

Military medicine can be called translational medicine or a branch of translational medicine. Using the methods of biology, pathophysiology, targeting pharmacology, pharmacological genetic phenotyping, and genetic phenotyping, military medicine can introduce new theories, concepts, and technology into basic research areas, such as epidemiology, pathogenesis and pathological response, mechanisms of complications after injury, regeneration after severe organ damage, mental stress, and psychological responses to somatic and mental trauma. The ultimate goal is to provide services in detection, prevention, diagnosis, and treatment.

Sanitary science and prevention medicine in extreme environments and in special military operation fields

Military activities, such as guarding, training, fighting, and surviving, are usually performed in special environments. The environment plays an important role in the health of military staff. The environment can refer to a natural environment (such as remote mountain areas, tropical areas, highlands, oceans, deserts, epidemic or space areas); human-made environments (such as closed, high-pressure, weightless environments); information environments (space fields with information or information-related launching, transmitting, utilizing media carriers); and mental environments (mental stress and mental health-related). Special operations should also include tasks in space, aviation, navigation, and underwater diving. The damage to humans in these areas is usually multi-factorial and more complicated and serious than single-factor damage.

For historical reasons, high-altitude-related military medical research is the strong point in Chinese military medicine, with many accomplished projects, such as the study of the effect and recovery of systemic or organic hypoxia and the mechanism of diseases on the plateau. More than 10 diagnostic criteria and management guidelines for high-altitude reactions and hypoxia coma have been developed, as well as a high-altitude standard sanitary system. In addition, military aviation medicine was established in 1949. Many types of aviation medical equipment have been developed by the military service in China in relation to much basic and applied research into mental health, aviation physiological training, pilot selection and unhealthy effects from hazardous aviation environments. Since the space program in China was established more than 40 years ago, aviation medical-engineering technology has rapidly developed and now has more than 13 branches, including aviation environmental medicine, cell biology, and psychiatry. A few branches, such as cardiology, have remained in a leading position in the world; however, some branches, such as aviation environment and psychiatry, remain behind the international level.

For military operations under a full-dimension environment, military medicine in China is now expanding its role in the field, reinforcing research into the military environment and into human-machine cooperation. Military medical research will potentiate the capability of human effectiveness and endurance under special situations and operations, including physical fitness, skillfulness, intelligence, human-machine cooperation, emotional perception and overall military operational capability, as well as survival in extreme environments and the enhancement of initiatives.

Preventing and managing injuries due to high-technology and new-concept weapons

Because of the rapid development of high-technology, new-concept, and special weapons, the prevention and management of injuries from these weapons are essential for military medicine. New-concept weapons have new injury mechanisms beyond traditional ones. Revolutionized weapons can also increase the range of human post-traumatic response, creating more difficult and complicated situations for treatment. In the research areas of damage from nuclear, chemical, and biological weapons and of secondary injury from these weapons, China has established standard "triple-prevention" rescue guidelines, including equipment and basic rescue techniques. In the area of detecting, preventing and managing microbiological agents, military medical research in China has reached the international level but should continue developing specialized military supply systems with minimal side effects. However, because of the restrictions in international law and arms control, the possibility of nuclear, chemical, and biological weapons being used is small. Sub-nuclear weapons (uranium bombs, powerful fuel air explosives, electromagnetic pulse weapons, deep penetrator weapons, and metal hydrogen weapons) or fourth-generation sub-nuclear, sub-chemical, and sub-biological weapons (such as incapacitating agents and detonation inhibitors) will bring about more healthcare problems.

Military medicine in China will continue to research the prevention and management of injuries caused by high-technology, new-concept and newly developed nuclear and chemical weapons. Injuries from these weapons include pathophysiological, serious, multi-organ, multi-location, combined, direct and indirect injuries as well as diseases during wartime; secondary psychiatric trauma and somatic trauma complicated with psychiatric trauma. Simultaneously, military medicine has to accelerate research into medical rescue, the production of presentational drugs, storage, equipment, and fast-detecting equipment and build up the basic laboratory research platform.

Military epidemiology

Epidemiologic prevention is an important field in military medicine. Military staffs are to be treated as a special group, with a close association with not only diseases in the entire country and society but also characteristics of confined living conditions, a rapidly changing population and extreme living conditions, such as remote mountains and oceans. The pathologies of such staffs greatly differ from those of the general population, particularly in terms of epidemiologic incidence and spread. In terms of biological and microbiological attacks, epidemiologic diseases will spread quickly. In addition to hard work in regular healthcare, researchers have to reinforce research into epidemiological prevention to prevent major outbreaks of diseases during or after war.

Recently, with the development of the military health care system, cooperation, wide application of new materials, new technologies, and the adoption of new standards, military medicine has developed research into new equipment and reforming tasks. Much large health equipment, such as sanitary trains, airplanes and war-zone hospitals, appeared in the healthcare and supply competition in 2009 to connect highways, railroads, and air medical rescue transportation and to establish a full-dimension new supply system, further improving the supply and support system. Six healthcare support systems were created: emergency rescue, full-dimension transportation, the prevention of nuclear-biological weapons, rapid response, and healthcare information technology and environmental protection under special situations. The largest navy hospital warship, "Peace Ark[2]," which was equipped with an ambulance boat, escort helicopter, and shipboard medical modular, established a modern medical treatment and rescue platform on the ocean for systemic search and rescue, management, and transportation. By connecting information technology between the land, sea, and air, a full-dimension healthcare system has been established with high-level technology and information and improvements from single to multiple elements, from loose-constructed to integrated construction, and from equipped mobile to mobile-equipped.

Currently, the efficiency and quality of the epidemiological surveillance system still needs to be improved. Simultaneously, scientists should accumulate experience in preventing epidemiological diseases adapted to preventive medicine's theory and technology system to help the public and to form the basis for future military medical activities. From the requirements for healthcare equipment from modern war, scientists need to upgrade the capacity of the supply system. In the future, the multi-functional and modular system must focus on improving the emergency-response mobile capacity, with the function of improved intellectualization, information, and mimicking war zones.

Information and networked healthcare system

With fast-developing Internet technology, newly developed practical, high-efficiency, and full-dimension information technology will be the priorities of the military medical information technology system. Digitalized medical information technology has been popularized at each level of the military system. By learning from developed countries and taking the actual military situation in China into account, military medicine has begun to build its own medical information system, with military characteristics, serving its modern national defense system and with the ability to win any regional war. In 1988, the General Hospital of PLA held its first clinical-case telephone conference with a hospital in Germany. Currently, the number of satellite telecommunication systems has exceeded 90, including telecommunications in Tibet, Xinjiang, and Xisha, which are remote areas. Each large military district has built a telecommunications center in the central and regional district hospitals and in basic medical clinics, as well as a telecommunications working station on ocean research vessels, which have completed many tasks including medical services in the first manned flight of Shenzhou in 2000.

Future war will have multiple levels and exchange and will bring more difficulties to the military supply system. How to immediately transport injured military staff to the hospital behind the frontline, which has life-saving capabilities and many military medical experts, is an important issue. Because of the variety of military tasks, many army forces have to live in remote areas, such as mountains, oceans, and islands under harsh living conditions. With the development of digitalized information technology, many medical resources can be shared with those remote areas, thus diminishing the differences between the remote areas and large cities and helping doctors and medical services with high-level medical equipment and experts.

Combining high-technology and traditional medicine in military medicine

New developments, such as genetic, cell, enzyme, and protein engineering, as well as genetic-chip, space-information, and nanometer technology, will bring rapid development for medical research. Development in neuron injury, space medicine, biology, radiology and radiation injury will provide important tools for military medicine research. These new developments can help lay new foundations for military medicine, establish new research models, and accomplish many special tasks in a new situation. These advanced and new technologies will orient military medicine toward diagnosis and treatment as well as toward detection and prevention. The establishment of mimicked human technology and military medical biological engineering will provide practical methods for researching medical rescue, medical assistance, the maintenance of the health of armed forces, and the enhancement of the effectiveness of the army supply system and for increasing the military capacity of armed forces.

Biotechnology can create new improvements in life information resources, micro-space and bio-control technology, involving the most important military information, such as ethnic genetic coding, functional control key, and creating new battling territory, with the ability of direct application to military defense attack systems and having "micro, defined, not lethal, and reversible" characteristics. Biotechnology can target changes in micro-structures and further define the control of special physiological functions to limit the injury of biological targets without lethal effects. Medical research into these issues can help develop military medicine.

Under the current requirements for military drug research and national medical strategy, scientists and doctors should disseminate the knowledge of traditional medicine among every level of the military forces. Scientists and doctors should find and develop military drugs from traditional medicine and must improve the survival ability of soldiers and officers, maintaining their mental health and combat force and improving military medical storage strategies. Using modern pharmacological research methods, such as molecular biology, molecular pharmacology, bio-neurology, bio-physics, cell biology, natural medical chemistry and computer science, scientists should increase the intensity of research into traditional medicine, focusing on selecting traditional drugs that meet the requirements of modern war.

Summary

Establishing a policy of military medicine is the guarantee of the new military medicine environment and revolutionized system. Establishing and completing military medical policy will push military medicine into the correct direction of scientific development. Scientists should base their policy on the requirements of future war, through appropriate cooperation with civilian research resources, emphasizing the selection and education of a special military medical branch, with deepening and widening directions. Scientists must rely on national resources in developed and advantaged areas to widen the range of military medical research with full-dimension development. To lay a solid foundation for future medical research, more military or civilian researchers and experts are needed.

(This article is excerpted from "Military medicine in China: old topic, new concept" published in *Military Medical Research*, PMID: 25722861)

Notes

1. the Gulf of Aden: an extension of the Indian Ocean, tucked between the Arabian Peninsula and the African continent. The gulf connects the Red Sea to the Arabian Sea. It has a long history as part of the Erythraean Sea and a critical oil shipping route linking the Far East and Europe. It is also a critical part of the Suez Canal shipping route, which connects the Red Sea and the Mediterranean Sea. 亚丁湾

2. Peace Ark： a large ship, 583 feet long and displacing at least 10,000 tons fully loaded. The ship is based with the South Sea Fleet at Zhoushan, in Zhejiang Province. While not underway, the ship normally has a crew of 113 and a medical complement of 20; on deployment those numbers increase to roughly 328 crew and 100 medical personnel. 和平方舟

Words and Expressions

1. somatic： *adj.* of or related to the body, especially as distinct from the mind 与躯体有关的

2. potentiate: *v.* to make effective or active 增强

3. perception: *n.* the way you notice things, especially with the senses 知觉；感知

4. revolutionize: *v.* to cause great changes in the way that it is done 彻底改变

5. secondary: *adj.* happening as a result of something else（疾病、感染等）间接引发的；继发性的

6. diminish: *v.* to become or to make something become smaller, weaker, etc. 减少；（使）减弱，（使）缩减

7. mimick: *v.* to try to be like somebody or something else 模仿

8. lethal: *adj.* causing or able to cause death 致命的；可致死的

9. disseminate: *v.* to spread information, knowledge, etc. so that it reaches many people 散布，传播（信息、知识等）

Medical Vocabulary

epidemiological disease: 流行病学疾病

pathophysiology: 病理生理学

targeting pharmacology: 靶向药理

genetic phenotyping: 基因表现型

pathogenesis: 发病机制

multi-factorial: 多基因（遗传）的

hypoxia:（组织）缺氧

aviation physiological training: 航空生理训练

electromagnetic pulse weapon：电磁脉冲武器

incapacitating agent：失能剂；失能性毒剂

detonation inhibitor：防爆剂

shipboard medical modular：船用医疗模块

enzyme：酶

protein engineering：［生化］蛋白质工程

nanometer technology：纳米技术

neuron：神经元；神经单位

bio-control technology：生物防治技术

Exercise

Critical Thinking

Military medicine is important in times of both war and peace. In this article, the author summarized the status quo and achievements in military medicine in China and described its future development. Though military medicine is an old topic, it is experiencing changes in the new era. Please discuss with your partner what challenges are facing your sphere of research and what you think can be done to cope with the situation.

Supplementary Reading

For more information on UN Peacekeeping, please go to the following websites:

1. https://peacekeeping.un.org/en

2. https://www.unmissions.org/

3. https://police.un.org/en

Unit Two UN Medical Support Structure

Text A
Medical Support in Peacekeeping Operations

The United Nations medical support mission is to secure the health and well-being of members of United Nations peacekeeping operations through planning, co-ordination, execution, monitoring and professional supervision of excellent medical care in the field.

1. Structure and Organization

There is a clear command structure within a peacekeeping force, with the most senior medical officer in the Mission, the Force Medical Officer (FMedO)[1], subordinated directly to the Force Commander (FC)[2] or the designated Head of Mission. The FMedO acts on behalf of the Force Commander on all medical matters and controls all UN field medical units providing Force-wide coverage. He also exercises professional supervision over organic medical units attached to their national contingents, which remain under the command of their respective Unit Commanders. Similarly, he seeks professional supervision from the MSD[3] and MSU[4] at UNHQ[5] on policy and operational matters respectively. These agencies work closely to ensure effective medical support for the Mission.

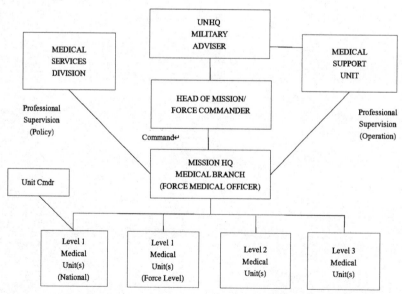

Figure 2-1 UN Medical Support Organization

2. UN Levels of Medical Support

Levels of medical support for UN peacekeeping missions have been standardized. This is necessary to ensure that the highest standards of medical care are provided to peacekeepers, particularly as medical units and personnel can come from different countries with varying standards of medical care. These levels are as follows:

2.1 Basic Level

This effectively refers to basic First Aid and preventive medicine practised at the smallest sub-unit level. As there is no doctor present, care is provided by the peacekeeper, or by a trained paramedic or nurse, using basic medical equipment and supplies. A summary of the training and equipping requirements can be found below.

Table 2-1   Basic Level Medical Support

TREATMENT CAPABILITY	TREATMENT CAPACITY	EQUIPMENT REQUIREMENT	REMARKS
-First Aid by non-medical personnel or paramedic - Core skills: 1. Cardiopulmonary resuscitation 2. Haemorrhage control 3. Fracture immobilisation 4. Wound dressing (including burns) 5. Casualty transport and evacuation 6. Communications and reporting		-First Aid Kit -Personal field dressing -Pocket mask (optional)	-Troop-contributing country to prepare peacekeepers with the required medical skills. -Peacekeepers to be trained in accordance with standards stipulated by MSU.

2.2 Level One Medical Support

This is the first level where a doctor is available. It provides first line primary health care, emergency resuscitation, stabilization and evacuation of casualties to the next level of medical care within a peacekeeping mission.

Tasks of a Level One Medical Unit:

a) Provide primary health care to a peacekeeping force of up to 700 in strength, with at least 20 ambulatory patients per day.

b) Conduct entry medical examination for peacekeepers if this has not already been done, and arrange for any necessary investigations.

c) Perform minor surgical procedures under local anaesthesia, e.g. toilet and suture of wounds, excision of lumps.

d) Perform emergency resuscitation procedures such as maintenance of airway and breathing, control of hemorrhage and treatment of shock.

e) Triage, stabilize and evacuate a casualty to the next level of medical care.

f) Ward up to 5 patients for up to 2 days each, for monitoring and inpatient treatment.

g) Administer vaccinations and other disease prophylaxis measures required in the mission area.

h) Perform basic field diagnostic and laboratory tests.

i) Maintain the capability to split into separate Forward Medical Teams (FMTs) to provide medical support simultaneously in two locations.

j) Oversees implementation of preventive medicine measures for the contingents and personnel under their care.

A Level One medical unit is to have adequate medical supplies and consumables for up to 60 days. Further details on the capabilities, staffing, equipping and infrastructural requirements of a Level One unit can be found below.

Table 2-2　Level One Medical Support

TREATMENT CAPABILITY	TREATMENT CAPACITY	MANPOWER REQUIREMENT	EQUIPMENT REQUIREMENT	INFRASTRUCTURE
1. Treatment of common illnesses 2. Advanced life support - airway maintenance - ventilation - haemorrhage control - treatment of shock and dehydration 3. Trauma management - fracture immobilisation - wound & burns management - infection control - analgesia	- Treatment of 20 ambulatory patients per day - Holding capacity of 5 patients for up to 2 days - Medical supplies & consumables for up to 60 days	2 x Medical Officer 6 x Paramedic/Nurse 3 x Support Staff NB: Capability of splitting into 2 x FMTs, each with 1 doctor and 2-3 paramedics	-Resuscitation and life support equipment, fluids and drugs -Field dispensary -Clinic and ward equipment set -Surgical sets for minor surgical procedures -Splints, bandages and stretchers -Portable doctor and paramedic bags/kits -Basic field laboratory kit -Sterilization equipment & refrigerator -1-2 x Ambulance	-Tentages or containers -Building (if available) -Basic general support and office facilities

2.3 Level Two Medical Support

This is the next level of medical care and the first level where surgical expertise and facilities are available. The mission of a Level Two medical facility is to provide second line health care, emergency resuscitation and stabilization, limb and life-saving surgical interventions, basic dental care and casualty evacuation to the next echelon.

Tasks of a Level Two Medical Unit:

a) Provide primary health care to a peacekeeping force of up to 1,000 in strength, with the capacity of treating up to 40 ambulatory patients per day.

b) Conduct entry and routine medical examination for peacekeepers if this is required, including any necessary investigations.

c) Perform limb and life-saving surgery such as laparotomy, appendectomy, thoracocentesis, wound exploration and debridement, fracture fixation and amputation. This must have the capacity to perform 3-4 major surgical procedures under general anesthesia per day.

d) Perform emergency resuscitation procedures such as maintenance of airway, breathing and circulation and advanced life support, hemorrhage control, and other life and limb saving emergency procedures.

e) Triage, stabilize and evacuate casualties to the next echelon of medical care.

f) Hospitalize up to 20 patients for up to seven days each for in-patient treatment and care, including intensive care monitoring for 1-2 patients.

g) Perform up to 10 basic radiological (X-ray) examinations per day.

h) Treat up to 10 dental cases per day, including pain relief, extractions, fillings and infection control.

i) Administer vaccinations and other disease prophylaxis measures as required in the mission area.

j) Perform up to 20 diagnostic laboratory tests per day, including basic hematology, blood biochemistry and urinalysis.

k) Constitute and deploy at least 2 FMTs (comprising 1 x doctor and 2 x paramedics) to provide medical care at secondary locations or medical support during land and air evacuation.

l) Maintain adequate medical supplies and consumables for up to 60 days, and the capability to resupply Level One units in the Mission area, if required.

Details on the capabilities, capacity, manpower and equipping requirements of a Level Two unit are shown below.

Table 2-3   Level Two Medical Support

TREATMENT CAPABILITY	TREATMENT CAPACITY	MANPOWER REQUIREMENT	EQUIPMENT REQUIREMENT	INFRASTRUCTURE
1. Treatment of common medical conditions	-Up to 40 outpatient visits per day	2 x Surgeons (general & orthopedic)	- Clinic and ward equipment	1. Hospital
2. Triage	-3 to 4 major surgeries	1 x Anaesthetist	- Resuscitation	- Reception / Admin
3. Advanced lifesupport and intensive care	per day	1 x Internist	room equipment	- Resuscitation room
4. Life and limb-saving surgery under anaesthesia	-10 to 20 inpatients for up to 7 days each	1 x General Physician	- Standard	- Outpatient consultation rooms
5. Pharmacy	- 5 to 10 dental	1 x Dentist	operating room	- 1-2 wards
6. Basic dental care	treatments per day	1 x Hygiene Officer	fixtures and	- 1-2 bed ICU
7. Basic laboratory facility	- 10 X-rays and 20	1 x Pharmacist	equipment	- Operating room
- Blood group & cross matching	laboratory tests per	1 x Head Nurse	- Intensive care	- Pharmacy
- Hemotology	day	2 x Intensive care nurses	equipment	- X-ray section
- Gram staining	- Medical supplies	1 x OT Assistant	- Field laboratory	- Laboratory section
- Blood film	and consumables for	10 x Nurses/Paramedic	and radiography	- Dental section
-Urinanalysis	60 days	1 x Radiographer	facility	- Sterilization area
8. Basic diagnostic radiography		1 x Laboratory technician	- Dental chair and equipment	2. Support Services
9. Hygiene control and preventive medicine		1 x Dental Assistant	- Hospital support	- Kitchen
10. Casualty evacuation to Level 3 or 4		2 x Drivers	equipment, e.g.	- Laundry
		8 x Support staff	autoclave, fridge	- Storage facility
		Total: 35	- 2 x Ambulance	- Maintenance facility
				- Communications
				- Generator
				- Office
				- Sanitation & waste disposal
				- Accommodation & messing

2.4 Level Three Medical Support

This is the highest level of medical care provided by a deployed UN medical unit. It combines the capabilities of Level One and Level Two units, with the additional capability of providing specialized in-patient treatment and surgery, as well as extensive diagnostic services. It is important to note that a Level Three unit is rarely deployed, and that this level of support is generally obtained from existing civilian or military hospitals within the Mission area or in a neighboring country.

Tasks of a Level Three Medical Unit:

a) Provide primary health care to a peacekeeping force of up to 5,000 in strength, with the capacity to treat up to 60 ambulatory patients per day.

b) Provide specialist medical consultation services, particularly in areas like Internal Medicine, Infectious Diseases, Tropical Medicine, Dermatology, Psychiatry and Gynaecology.

c) Perform up to 10 major general and orthopedic surgical procedures under general anesthesia per day. Availability of specialist surgical disciplines (e.g. neurosurgery, cardiothoracic surgery, trauma surgery, urology, burns unit) is an advantage.

d) Perform emergency resuscitation procedures such as maintenance of airway, breathing and circulation and advanced life support.

e) Stabilize casualties for long-haul air evacuation to a Level 4 facility, which may be located in another country.

f) Hospitalize up to 50 patients for up to 30 days each for inpatient treatment and care, and up to 4 patients for intensive care and monitoring.

g) Perform up to 20 basic radiological (X-ray) examinations per day. Availability of ultra-sonography or CT scan capability is an advantage.

h) Treat 10-20 dental cases per day, including pain relief, extractions, fillings and infection control, as well as limited oral surgery.

i) Administer vaccination and other preventive medicine measures, including vector control in the Mission area.

j) Perform up to 40 diagnostic laboratory tests per day.

k) Constitute and deploy at least two FMTs (comprising 1 x doctor and 2 x paramedics) to provide medical care at secondary locations or medical support during casualty evacuation by land, rotary and fixed-wing aircraft.

l) Maintain adequate medical supplies and consumables for up to 60 days, and the capability of limited resupply Level One and Level Two medical units, if required.

Details on the capabilities, manpower, equipment and infrastructural requirements for a Level Three facility is shown below.

Table 2-4   Level Three Medical Support

TREATMENT CAPABILITY	TREATMENT CAPACITY	MANPOWER REQUIREMENT	EQUIPMENT REQUIREMENT	INFRASTRUCTURE
All capabilities of Level Two facility. In addition: 1. Specialist consultation services 2. Multi-discipline surgical services 3. Post-operative & intensive care 4. Full laboratory services 5. Diagnostic radiology, ideally with ultrasound & CT-scan 6. Pharmacy 7. Dental surgery and X-ray	- Up to 60 outpatient visits per day - Up to 10 major surgeries per day - Up to 50 inpatients for up to 30 days each - 10-20 dental treatments per day - 20 X-rays and 40 laboratory tests per day - Medical supplies and consumables for 60 days	16 x Doctors - General surgeons - Orthopedic surgeon - Anaesthetists - Internists - General physician - Dermatologist - Psychiatrist - Other specialists 1 x Dental Surgeon 1 x Dentist 2 x Dental Asst 1 x Hygiene Officer 1 x Pharmacist 1 x Pharmacist Assistant 50 x Nursing staff - Head nurses - ICU nurses - OR Assistants - Nurses - Paramedics 2 x Radiographer 2 x Lab technician 14 x Support staff Total: 91	As for Level Two facility. In addition: - OR fixtures and equipment for general surgery & orthopedics - Intensive and highdependency care equipment - Laboratory and radiography equipment - Dental chairs and X-ray - Ambulances - General transport	1. Hospital - Reception/Admin - Resuscitation room - 4 x Outpatient consultation room - 2-4 x Ward - 4-bed ICU - 2 x Operating room - Pharmacy - X-ray unit - Laboratory unit - Dental surgery (2 chair) - Dental X-ray room - Sterilization room 2. Support Services - Kitchen - Laundry - Storage facility - Maintenance facility - Communications - Generators - Fuel store - Water purification - Sanitation and waste disposal - Accommodation & messing

2.5 Level Four Medical Support

A Level Four medical facility provides definitive medical care and specialist medical treatment unavailable or impractical to provide within a Mission area. This includes specialist surgical and medical procedures, reconstruction, rehabilitation and convalescence. Such treatment is highly specialized and costly, and may be required for a long duration. It is neither practical nor cost-effective for the UN to deploy such a unit within the Mission area. Such services are generally sought in the host country, a neighboring country, or in the troop-contributing country itself. The UN can arrange transfer of a patient or casualty to such a facility, and for reasons of cost, compensation and pension, continue to monitor the patient's progress.

Indications for UN medical staff to utilize Level 4 facilities include:

a) When the distance from the Mission area to the country of origin is too far, and the patient or casualty is in urgent need of specialist medical treatment.

b) When the patient requires only short-term specialist treatment and is expected to return to duty within 30 days.

c) When the troop-contributing country is unable to provide appropriate definitive treatment (this excludes chronic medical conditions diagnosed prior to the peacekeeper's deployment into the Mission area, or for which he is already receiving treatment).

d) When the UN receives an offer from a specific nation to provide definitive care, an arrangement requiring a contract or Letter of Assist (LOA)[6] with the respective country and allocation of the appropriate funds.

2.6 Forward Medical Team

A Forward Medical Team (FMT) is a small, highly mobile medical unit of about 3 men that is configured and equipped to provide short-term medical support in the field. This is generally constituted as and when required from existing medical units within the Mission area (including personnel, equipment and supplies), but may be a separate entity requested from troop-contributing countries and deployed with an independent mission. FMTs depend on the units they support for all service support requirements.

Tasks of a Forward Medical Team:

a) To provide primary healthcare and emergency medical services at a medical post supporting an isolated military contingent of about 100-150 personnel.

b) To provide first line medical support for short-term field operations in areas without immediate access to UN medical facilities.

c) To provide continuous medical care during land and/or air evacuation of casualties particularly for seriously ill or unstable casualties, and where evacuation distances are long or where delays are anticipated. This includes medical evacuation out of the Mission area into a nearby country or medical repatriation, if indicated.

d) To provide a medical team for Search and Rescue missions.

To function effectively in the above operations, it is important for FMTs to be well equipped despite their size, including the requirement for life-support medical equipment. All equipment and supplies need to be portable and configured for use in confined spaces like ambulances and helicopters.

(This article is excerpted from *Medical Support Manual for United Nations Peacekeeping Operations, 2nd Edition*)

Notes

1. the Force Medical Officer (FMedO): In an integrated civilian-military mission, the FMedO is the most senior ranking military medical officer within the peacekeeping force and the medical adviser to the Force Commander on all military operational and tactical medical matters. 部队医务主任

2. the Force Commander (FC): the head of Mission in the UN peacekeeping operations who has operational control and responsibility to the missions designated by the UN 部队指挥官

3. the MSD: It refers to the Medical Services Division, which develops and promulgates medical support and health care polices for UN peacekeeping missions. 医务司

4. the MSU: It refers to the Medical Support Unit, which is the executive arm of the UN for planning, coordinating and monitoring medical support in the field. 医务股

5. the UNHQ: the United Nations Headquarters 联合国总部

6. Letter of Assist (LOA): a document issued by the UN to a government or agency, authorizing the provision of goods or services to a UN peacekeeping mission. Reimbursement will be made for the cost of the goods or services, as well as for depreciation value of equipment in accordance to agreed guidelines. 协助通知书

Words and Expressions

1. contingent: *n.* all formed units, personnel and equipment of the troop/police-contributor deployed to a mission area（维和行动）分队

2. stipulate: *v.* to state clearly and firmly that something must be done, or how it must be done 规定；明确要求

3. ambulatory: *adj.* able to walk about 能走动的，非卧床的

4. evacuate: *v.* to send someone to a place of safety, away from a dangerous building, town, or area 疏散；使……撤离

5. echelon: *n.* a formation of troops, ships, aircraft, or vehicles in parallel rows with the end of each row projecting further than the one in front（士兵、飞机等的）梯形编队，梯队

6. deploy: *v.* to organize or position troops or military resources so that they are ready to be used 部署

7. messing: *n.* the building at a military base or military barracks in which members of the armed forces can eat or relax（军队的）餐厅

8. prior to: something happens before a particular time or event 在……之前

9. allocation: *n.* an amount of something, especially money, that is given to a particular person or used for a particular purpose（尤指经费）配置；分配

10. configure: *v.* to set up a piece of computer equipment so that it is ready for us 配置（计算机设备）

11. repatriation: *n.* the act of returning to the country of origin 遣返

Medical Vocabulary

cardiopulmonary resuscitation: (abbr: CPR) 心肺复苏术
haemorrhage control: 止血
fracture immobilization: 骨折固定
dressing: 敷料
suture: 缝合
excision: 切除

lump: 肿块

prophylaxis: 疾病预防

shock: 休克

dehydration: 脱水

analgesia: 镇痛

medical supplies: 医用物资

consumables: 耗材

dispensary: 药房

splint: 夹板

bandage: 绷带

stretcher: 担架

sterilization: 消毒

tentage: 帐篷

container: 方舱

laparotomy: 剖腹术

appendectomy: 阑尾切除术

thoracocentesis: 胸腔穿刺术

debridement: 清创术

amputation: 截肢

anesthesia: 麻醉

extraction: 拔牙

filling: 补牙

basic hematology: 血常规

blood biochemistry: 血生化

urinalysis: 尿常规

paramedic: （医疗）护理人员，卫生员

orthopedic: 整形外科的

internist: 内科医生

autoclave: 高压灭菌器

dermatology: 皮肤病学

psychiatry: 精神病学

gynecology: 妇科学

vector control: 病媒控制

high dependency care equipment: 高依赖性监护设备

convalescence: 康复

Exercises

I. Reading Comprehension

A. Directions: Decide whether the following statements are True or False according to the text.

1. The FMedO controls all UN field medical units and their national units.

2. Medical units from different countries provide different standards of medical support for UN peacekeeping missions.

3. Medical care is usually provided by paramedics or nurses at the basic level.

4. Basic dental treatments can be obtained at the Level One medical unit.

5. A Level One medical unit has the capacity to provide medical support in one location.

6. A Level Two medical unit is the first level where surgical expertise and facilities are available.

7. If you need a basic hematology test, you have to go to a Level Two medical unit or above.

8. All levels of medical units possess medial supplies and consumables for up to 60 days.

9. Level Four medical support is the highest level of medical care provided by a deployed UN medical unit.

10. FMTs are separate entities which provide highly mobile medical support within the Mission area.

B. Directions: Answer the following questions according to your understanding of the text.

1. According to the text, who oversees all medical matters in UN peacekeeping operations?

2. What are the agencies that are directly involved with medical care for UN personnel?

3. Why is medical support divided into different levels for UN peacekeeping operations?

4. Who provides medical care at the smallest sub-unit level?

5. What is the treatment capability of a Level One medical unit?

6. Can you introduce the medical personnel requirements of a Level Two medical unit?

7. Which level is taken as the highest level of medical care provided by a deployed UN medical unit?

8. Why is a Level Four medical unit rare to see within a Mission area?

9. What requirements should be met for a Forward Medical Team to perform tasks effectively?

10. At what level(s) of a medical unit accommodations and messing are provided?

II. Vocabulary

Directions: Choose the best word or expression from the list given for each blank. Use each word or expression only once and make proper changes when necessary.

evacuate	stipulate	contingent	prior to
allocation	deploy	configure	repatriation

1. After you have successfully installed these products, you must next _____ demo environments.

2. A State Department spokeswoman said that the aid _____ for Pakistan was still under review.

3. The fire is threatening about sixty homes, and residents _____ the area.

4. Nigeria provided a large _____ of troops to the West African Peacekeeping Force.

5. Some laws also _____ in explicit terms that Chinese citizens have obligations to take care of parents and raise children.

6. _____ 200 B.C., a number of relatively small centers coexisted in and near the Valley of Mexico.

7. What is clear is that the _____ of capital has been painful for those countries that relied heavily on international capital flows.

8. At least 5,000 missiles _____ along the border.

III. Topics for Discussion

1. Please discuss with your partner the UN medical support structure based on Figure 2-1 in the text.

2. What other capabilities does a Level Three medical unit provide apart from the combination of Level One and Level Two units?

3. Choose any two levels of medical units and make a comparison in terms of treatment capacity, manpower and equipment requirement.

Text B
An Interview with UNFICYP's Force Medical Officer[1]

In times of COVID-19, the challenges facing peacekeeping missions around the world have multiplied, the health crisis has highlighted the key role of our medical teams in ensuring peacekeepers remain safe and healthy while continuing mission operations across the buffer zone[2]. Health professionals have been heroes during the past year and deserve our praise and thanks for the work they do to tackle the pandemic and keep us all safe. We talked to our Force Medical Officer, Lieutenant Colonel Gábor Kolonics from Hungary, who was deployed with UNFICYP in September 2020. Lieutenant Kolonics shared his experiences during pandemic, UNFICYP's approach and action plan to cope with the challenges posed by

COVID-19.

Can you give a brief overview of UNFICYP's COVID-19 pandemic action plan?

Our approach from day one has been rooted in science, working closely with the local authorities and ensuring all preventative measures are strictly adhered to by all our peacekeepers. UNFICYP's pandemic action plan has been designed and regularly updated according to the guidelines and experiences from the World Health Organization, the European Centre for Disease Prevention and Control[3] and following local administrations' guidelines from both communities on the island.

What major steps have been taken to improve internal communications on the spread of the pandemic from a medical point of view?

Sharing information timely and accurately has been the key to our plan of action. A proper chain of command is followed, and a dedicated COVID-19 response team keeps the chief medical officer appraised of the situation across the mission. In addition, a COVID-19 committee was established to keep the information chain connected from headquarters to all sectors and ensure information arrives in a timely manner. Under the command and leadership directives, the medical team has been vigilant to spread awareness for peacekeepers' safety and health through our medics across the Mission.

How are the sectors and unit-level commanders dealing with preventive measures to continue routine patrolling and their other duties?

I must say, the commanding officers of units and sectors are playing a key role in pushing the Mission directives through all ranks and through the chain of command and medical teams in the sectors. We have independent medical teams with doctors and staff in all sectors, this has enabled peacekeepers to continue their duties uninterrupted.

I am thankful to my complete medical team and to the support we received from the headquarters supply department, together with them we were able to spread information about preventive measures without compromising the operational capabilities and personal comfort of the peacekeepers.

What specific guidelines does the UN have for meetings and mass gatherings during this COVID-19 period?

The nature of the work performed by office staff at headquarters was mostly shifted to telecommuting. Whereas under operational requirements when physical interaction is necessary, it is done within the COVID-19 guidelines. Wearing of masks, physical distancing, following local administrations' preventive measures and UN guidelines is strictly followed. In addition, the concept of "teams within teams" is implemented in the working environment at every level in the sectors and sub-units at UNFICYP.

According to WHO, what routine cleaning and disinfection procedures are appropriate for containing the spread of COVID-19 that UNFICYP is following?

UNFICYP peacekeepers actively follow the mandate and for its enforcement a key part is patrolling the buffer zone. For this purpose, we follow all the basic worldwide preventive and precautionary measures and WHO's principles like the mandatory use of masks, regular cleaning of hands, disinfection of office areas and vehicles before and after patrolling and physical distancing. This way, the peacekeeping operation is not disturbed, and proper precautions are also catered for.

As a Force Medical Officer, what was the biggest challenge you experienced while serving at UNFICYP?

With COVID-19 we have experienced the situation changing on day-to-day basis, which requires regular information sharing, timely reporting and transparency. UNFICYP's medical team from headquarters and across the sectors are playing a vital role to meet up with these challenging times. Under the directions of leadership and medical science's roles and regulations we have tried our best to meet up every challenge and come out with a new learning for the way forward.

What would you like to say about the mental health and associated issues related with the pandemic and how peacekeepers have coped with it in UNFICYP?

I would say mental health is interconnected with the physical status and wellbeing of our personnel. It is not only during the current pandemic, but peacekeepers are recommended to keep themselves fit and mentally vigilant during the whole period they serve in the Mission. We have strongly recommended to peacekeepers, irrespective of the pandemic, to practice sports regularly, eat healthy, and most importantly, to avoid rumours and false information related with COVID-19 and UNFICYP has successfully carried out physical and military exercises during the pandemic.

What are the COVID-19 protocols being followed for the troop rotations?

UNFICYP undergoes regular biannual rotations across all sectors of the contingents and of individual staff officers without any disturbance to the operational requirement. We have been successful to cope with the COVID-19 pandemic environment and successfully carried out our rotation and are ready to go for first one of 2021 in next months. We apply all rules and regulations and in addition, we included a period of two-week quarantine for all new arrivals, a period which includes testing and following all necessary requirements before peacekeepers can start their duties. On the other hand, individual staff rotation continues throughout the year with newer procedures and arrangements from our support department we have been able to continue uninterrupted.

What are the most common myths about COVID-19 that you would dispel for patients?

There are several myths going online, for instance, we hear a lot of fake news related to the intake of vitamins and mineral supplements can cure COVID-19, the prolonged use of masks causes CO_2 intoxication or oxygen deficiency, extreme weather can kill the virus, antibiotics prevent or cure COVID-19 and these are just to name a few. I strongly discourage such myths, and during my interactions, I recommend to our peacekeepers not to overburden themselves with over-thinking. We can stay safe by following simple and straight measures under WHO guidelines to stop the spread of the virus.

In your opinion, how to save people's lives without compromising their livelihoods?

I believe there have been an overabundance of information, both online and offline. We must keep ourselves realistic and positive at the same time. Rationally acting upon the precautionary measures and keeping healthy is what is needed at the time. We all wish for a better and safer 2021.

(The full article is available at https://unficyp.unmissions.org/interview-unficyp%E 2%80%99s-force-medical-officer-g%C3%A1bor-kolonics)

Notes

1. UNFICYP: The United Nations Peacekeeping Force in Cyprus is a United Nations peacekeeping force that was originally set up by the Security Council in 1964 to prevent further fighting between the Greek Cypriot and Turkish Cypriot communities and to contribute to the maintenance and restoration of law and order and to facilitate a return to normal conditions. Major General Cheryl Pearce is the current Force Commander of UNFICYP, appointed in 2018, and preceded by Major General Mohammad Humayun Kabir. 联合国驻塞浦路斯维持和平部队

2. the buffer zone: It is formed to create an area of separation between disputing or belligerent forces and reduce the risk of renewed conflict, also called area of separation in some United Nations operations. 缓冲区

3. the European Centre for Disease Prevention and Control: an agency of the European Union whose mission is to strengthen Europe's defenses against infectious diseases. It covers a wide spectrum of activities, such as surveillance, epidemic intelligence, response, scientific advice, microbiology, preparedness, public health training, international relations, health communication, and the scientific journal *Eurosurveillance*. 欧洲疾病预防控制中心

Words and Expressions

1. adhere to: to stick firmly to something 遵守

2. appraise: *v.* to consider or examine somebody/something and form an opinion about them or it 估量；估价

3. vigilant: *adj.* very careful to notice any signs of danger or trouble 警觉的；警惕的

4. patrol: *n.* a group of soldiers or vehicles to go around an area or a building at regular times to check that it is safe and that there is no trouble 巡逻；巡查

5. compromise: *v.* to reach an agreement with others in which you both give up something that you originally wanted 妥协；折中

6. mandate: *n.* an official order given to someone to perform a particular task（个人所获

得的）授权

7. irrespective of: without considering something or being influenced by it 不考虑；不受……影响

8. quarantine: *n.* a period of time when an animal or a person that has or may have a disease is kept away from others in order to prevent the disease from spreading（为防传染的）隔离期；检疫

9. dispel: *v.* to make something, especially a feeling or belief, go away or disappear 驱散，消除（尤指感觉或信仰）

10. intoxication: *n.* the condition of having physical or mental control markedly diminished by the effects of alcohol or drugs 中毒

Exercise

Critical Thinking

Lieutenant Colonel Kolonics, UNFICYP's Force Medical Officer, shared his experiences and his team's work in coping with the challenges posed by the pandemic. Please summarize what measures they have taken to ensure the routine duties amid COVID-19 and discuss with your partner the possible preventive and protective advice you would like to give.

Supplementary Reading

For more information on UN Medical Support Structure, please go to the following websites:

1. http://repository.un.org/bitstream/handle/11176/387299/2015.12%20Medical%20Support%20Manual%20for%20UN%20Field%20Missions.pdf?sequence=4&isAllowed=y

2. http://dag.un.org/bitstream/handle/11176/387419/CopyofTCCGenericGuidelinesApprovedsigned7March2008.pdf?sequence=1&isAllowed=y

3. https://www.researchgate.net/publication/12885529_Levels_of_Medical_Support_for_United_Nations_Peacekeeping_Operations

Unit Three   Medical Treatment for UN Peacekeeping Operations

Text A
Casualty Treatment and Evacuation

1. Triage

Medical triage is the categorization of a patient or casualty based on clinical evaluation, for the purpose of establishing priorities for treatment and evacuation. This facilitates the effective use of limited medical resources and ensures the survival of the greatest possible number in a multiple casualty scenario. Triage is generally conducted by the most experienced doctor or paramedic. This is a continuous process as the casualty's condition may deteriorate, particularly during evacuation. It should be performed upon arrival at a medical facility and again, prior to evacuation for further treatment.

1.1 Classification

Different triage classifications have been adopted by international and national health care organizations. These categorize a patient or casualty according to the urgency for evacuation or treatment, taking into consideration his/her likely prognosis. Some systems are based on trauma scoring, while others depend primarily on clinical judgement. It is important for medical units to be familiar with the triage classification and tags of other units within a Mission area.

1.2 Triage Categories

The UN recommends adopting a 4-category triage nomenclature based on the severity of the medical condition and urgency for treatment.

a) Priority 1 (RED: Immediate). This category has the highest priority for treatment or evacuation, as urgent resuscitative interventions are required to ensure survival of the casualty or patient. Examples include airway obstruction, respiratory emergencies, shock and severe trauma. It is likely that such cases will die within 2 hours or earlier, in the absence of appropriate medical treatment.

b) Priority 2 (YELLOW: Urgent). This comprises cases that require early treatment, particularly surgery, and it is recommended that evacuation to a surgical facility take place within 6 hours of injury. Examples include visceral injury, closed thoracic injury without threatening asphyxia, major limb injuries and fractures, closed head injury, open eye injury and moderate burns.

c) Priority 3 (GREEN: Delayed or Hold). Treatment is less urgent in this category and can be deferred if there are other casualties requiring limited treatment or evacuation assets. Examples include simple closed fractures, soft tissue injury, closed chest injury and maxillary-facial injury.

d) Priority 4 (BLACK: Expectant or Deceased). This category refers to casualties whose injuries or illness are so serious that they have minimal chances of survival or who are dead on arrival. Should there be competition for limited medical resources, such cases will have lower priority for evacuation or treatment, despite the severity of their condition. Examples include brain-stem death and terminal illness.

2. Treatment and Holding Policy

2.1 Treatment available at a medical facility is determined by the level of medical support it provides. At the lower levels, the emphasis is on resuscitating a casualty and stabilizing him for evacuation to the next level. In serious injuries, definitive treatment is rarely available here and efforts should be made to minimize delaying subsequent evacuation.

2.2 The organization of medical resources within a Mission area is determined by the treatment and evacuation capability at each level. If difficulties or delays in evacuation are anticipated, these levels must correspondingly have greater treatment capability. The holding policy (also known as evacuation policy) within a Mission balances the treatment capability of each level against the availability of evacuation assets. This is achieved by stating the maximum period a patient may be treated at each level, following which he will be transferred if he cannot return to duty. This policy is determined by:

a) Limitations on evacuation caused by unavailability of evacuation assets, operational constraints, weather or topography.

b) Demand on medical resources, e.g. when large numbers of patients are anticipated, the holding duration may shorten.

c) Availability of medical assets, e.g. at the start or drawdown of a Mission, there are relatively little facilities and holding period is relatively short.

3. Medical Evacuation and Repatriation

3.1 The responsibility for planning and establishing an effective medical evacuation system lies with the planning staff in DPKO and the administration and medical staff in the Mission area. The FMedO co-ordinates all in-theatre evacuation activities, with the support of the Mission administration and the guidance of the Medical Services Division. Details of the evacuation plan are to be included within every Mission's Standard Operating Procedures (SOP)[1]. There are three categories of patient or casualty transfer, these being:

a) Casualty Evacuation (Casevac). Evacuation of a casualty from the site of injury to the closest medical facility, which should ideally be conducted within 1 hour of injury.

b) Medical Evacuation (Medevac). Evacuation of a casualty between two medical facilities, either within the Mission area (in-theatre) or out of it (out-of-theatre). The casualty may either return to duty (RTD) within the time-frame stipulated in the holding policy, or be repatriated.

c) Medical Repatriation. Return of a patient or casualty to his home-country because of medical reasons, following which he would be unlikely to return to duty.

3.2 Planning Determinants

a) Mission Holding Policy. As discussed above, a Mission holding policy has to be set from the onset of an operation, which dictates the maximum period (in days) a patient may be held at each level of medical care. This in turn determines the treatment capability and capacity required at each level and the supporting evacuation requirements.

b) Fitness for Evacuation. The clinical condition of a patient is the key criterion in determining timing and means of evacuation between levels of care.

c) Evacuation Time to Medical Facility. Evacuation must be conducted in a timely manner, allowing a patient requiring life or limb-saving intervention to receive this as early as possible. It is recommended that casualty evacuation to a Level 2 or 3 facility should take no more than 4 hours from the time of injury.

d) Air Evacuation. While not always possible, it is ideal to have dedicated helicopters for medical evacuation, manned by Forward Medical Teams equipped with essential life-support equipment and supplies. Should Level 2 and/or 3 support not be available within the Mission area, rotary or fixed-wing aircraft must be made available at short notice for Medevac to such facilities.

3.3 Medical Evacuation (Medevac)

Medevac will be considered when available local medical facilities are not adequate to provide the necessary treatment. Policies and procedures concerning Medevac are as follows:

a) Internationally recruited staff members, Military and Civilian personnel may be evacuated at United Nations' expense for the purpose of securing essential medical care or treatment not available within the Mission area. Locally recruited staff, their spouses and dependant children may be evacuated in emergency situations when the medical risk is very high or when a life-threatening condition is present.

b) In emergency situations, the Chief of the Mission or Force Commander may directly authorise medical evacuations, after consultation with the FMedO and the Chief Administration Officer (CAO)[2]. Prior approval by UNHQ is not required within the Mission area.

c) Evacuation may be by land or air transportation and should be to the closest appropriate medical facility to the duty station. The nature of illness or injury, the type of treatment required and the language spoken must also be taken into consideration. The use of dedicated means of transport clearly marked with the Red Cross/Red Crescent insignia is preferred.

d) It is essential that the patient's pre-evacuation and in-flight treatment is adequately documented and accompanies the patient to the next medical facility. If indicated, travel of an accompanying doctor or nurse may be authorized.

e) For childbirth, psychiatric conditions and illnesses requiring prolonged recuperation, medical evacuation to the place of home leave or repatriation to the home country should be encouraged.

f) Should a staff member prefer medical evacuation to his/her place of home leave, as opposed to the recommended place of evacuation, such travel may be authorized as advanced home leave.

g) Should a nation prefer to evacuate its own personnel contrary to the opinion of the medical officer in charge or the FMedO, it becomes a national responsibility and at the nation's expense.

h) In non-emergency cases, UNHQ approval is to be sought prior to Medevac. In emergencies, this is not required, although UNHQ is to be informed immediately after Medevac has taken place. These are to be submitted to the Field Administration and Logistics Division (FALD) [3] and the UN Medical Director [4].

i) After having been certified fit by the attending doctor, a copy of the certificate should be forwarded to the Director, MSD, who will either approve or deny return to the duty station. In cases of serious illness or injury, the patient may not return to duty at UN cost prior to approval by the Medical Director. This does not apply for non-emergency cases.

j) Procedures for Medevac of Military personnel must be detailed in the Standing Operations Procedure (SOP) for the Mission. Guidelines for Medevac of UN staff are outlined in the UN Field Administration Manual, while further details can be found in the Revised ST/AI on Medical Evacuation.

3.4 Medical Repatriation

Medical repatriation is evacuation of a patient or casualty back to his/her country or parent duty station. Policies and procedures concerning repatriation are as follows:

a) Repatriation on medical grounds apply to all personnel who are unlikely to be fit to return to duty based on the holding policy (evacuation policy) established, or who require treatment not available within the Mission area. In general, 30 days is the accepted guideline for holding policy.

b) Medical repatriation is the responsibility of the FMedO, in co-ordination with the respective national contingent commander and the Chief Administration Officer (CAO). Once an individual is repatriated, further medical care is a national responsibility.

c) Military personnel arriving in the Mission area who are unfit for duty will be repatriated immediately at the nation's expense. If repatriation is required for a chronic medical condition diagnosed or under treatment at the time of Mission assignment, expenses may have to be borne by the Troop Contributing Country.

d) Pregnant women should be repatriated by the end of the fifth month of gestation.

e) All personnel with clinical symptoms or signs of AIDS must be repatriated.

f) Authorization for repatriation must be obtained in advance from the Director, Medical Services Division. A written recommendation must be submitted by the FMedO or doctor in charge, regardless of whether costs are to be borne by the UN, a national government or the individual concerned. Once authorized, the CAO proceeds to arrange repatriation by the Mission or contingent via the most economical means.

g) If possible, regular rotation or scheduled service flights should be utilized for repatriation. Payment of travel subsistence allowance and terminal expenses may be authorized in cases undertaken at UN expense, and baggage allowance is identical to that of personnel rotated on an individual basis. Should an escort be required, this is limited to the free allowance granted by the airline and in accordance to existing rules and regulations.

h) For cases requiring urgent medical repatriation, military or civilian aircraft may be contracted. The UN has since 1989 maintained a standing arrangement with the Government of Switzerland regarding air ambulance services for peacekeeping operations. These services are provided by La Garde Aerienne Suisse de Sauvetage (REGA) [5]. It has to be noted that REGA provides medical staff and equipment during the evacuation.

4. Mass Casualty and Disaster Management

This section refers specifically to situations involving UN personnel, while the provision of humanitarian assistance to the local population will be considered separately. All medical units have to prepare for mass casualty situations and disasters within the Mission area. Contingencies must be planned and resources allocated at the beginning of a new mission, and co-ordinated in line with the Mission's operational and security plans. Plans should be prepared at each level, from the Team Site through the Contingent HQ, Sector HQs and up to Mission HQ level.

4.1 Definition

A mass casualty situation or disaster is a temporary situation, during which insufficient resources are available to manage the multiple casualties, thereby increasing the likelihood of morbidity and death. This can be the result of a natural or manmade catastrophe, and may be accompanied by substantial material damage to infrastructure and environment.

4.2 Medical Support

a) In the acute phase, medical units will mobilize all their available resources to provide immediate support. This includes establishing First Aid posts and Medical Regulation Centers at the incident site, as well as to support search and rescue activities.

b) Triage is important here to establish priority for treatment, and for evacuation by land and air to UN, local and NGO medical facilities. It is essential that evacuation of casualties to these facilities is centrally co-ordinated and managed.

c) Treatment provided at the site should be limited to Basic Life Support and casualty resuscitation. The primary objective is stabilization of the injured and their evacuation to adequately staffed and equipped medical facilities.

d) Brief documentation of casualty data, injuries and treatment provided should accompany all casualties. If available, triage tags should be attached.

e) Managing the dead should be planned, including on-site identification (if possible). Close co-operation with the local administration is required to ensure smooth handling and transfer of remains for definitive identification and burial.

4.3 Planning Guidelines

a) Identifying risk factors and potential threats, including hostile acts by local parties.

b) Preparing inventory of available medical resources within the Mission area, including evacuation assets and local infrastructure.

c) Contingency planning to include grouping of medical units, defining areas of responsibility and individual tasks, identifying potential casualty holding areas and evacuation routes.

d) Forming Ops Center to centralize medical resource allocation and co-ordination of evacuation.

e) Communications plan including allocation of radio resources and co-ordination with other UN agencies, national authorities and NGOs.

f) Logistics support, including medical supplies.

g) Special medical requirements, including medical debriefing[6] and stress management of victims, rescue and medical personnel.

(This article is excerpted from *Medical Support Manual for United Nations Peacekeeping Operations, 2nd Edition*)

Notes

1. Standard Operating Procedures (SOP): a set of step-by-step instructions compiled by an organization to help workers carry out routine operations. SOPs aim to achieve efficiency, quality output and uniformity of performance, while reducing miscommunication and failure to comply with industry regulations. 标准作业程序

2. Chief Administration Officer (CAO): a top-tier executive who supervises the daily operations of an organization and is ultimately responsible for its performance（维和行动）首席行政干事

3. the Field Administration and Logistics Division (FALD): one of the two sections belonging to the Office of Planning and Support 后勤司

4. UN Medical Director: a physician who provides guidance and leadership on the use of medicine in a healthcare organization 联合国医疗司司长

5. La Garde Aerienne Suisse de Sauvetage (REGA): Swiss Air-Rescue is a private, non-profit air rescue service that provides emergency medical assistance in Switzerland and

Liechtenstein. REGA was established in 1952 and mainly assists with mountain rescues. REGA also provides a repatriation and medical advice service for members who experience a medical emergency while abroad and local treatment is not available. 瑞士空中救援队

6. medical debriefing: sometimes held after a significant event, such as a particularly difficult resuscitation or a mass causality incident. The concept of debriefings was started by the military. Debriefings were held after a mission to develop better strategies and allow soldiers a chance to talk about what occurred and process the events. 医疗情况汇报

Words and Expressions

1. deteriorate: *v.* to become worse in some way 恶化

2. evacuation: *n.* the action or process of withdrawing from a place in an organized way especially for protection 撤离，疏散

3. nomenclature: *n.* a system of naming things, especially in a branch of science（尤指某学科的）命名法

4. defer: *v.* to arrange for an event or action to happen at a later date, rather than immediately or at the previously planned time 推迟

5. anticipate: *v.* to see what might happen in the future and take action to prepare for it 预见，预计（并做准备）

6. topography: *n.* the physical features of an area of land, especially the position of its rivers, mountains, etc. 地形；地貌

7. drawdown: *n.* a depletion or reduction, for example of supplies 削减

8. dictate: *v.* to tell somebody what to do, especially in an annoying way（尤指以令人不快的方式）指使，强行规定

9. insignia: *n.* a design or symbol that shows that a person or object belongs to a particular organization, often a military one 徽章

10. recuperation: *n.* the process or period of gradually regaining one's health and strength 恢复；复原

11. hostile: *adj.* (to/towards somebody/something) very unfriendly or aggressive and ready to argue or fight 敌意的；敌对的

Medical Vocabulary

resuscitative intervention: 复苏干预
airway obstruction: 气道阻塞
visceral injury: 脏器损伤
thoracic: 胸的
asphyxia: 窒息
maxillary-facial: 颌面的
brain-stem death: 脑干死亡

gestation: 妊娠

Exercises

I. Reading Comprehension

A. Directions: Decide whether the following statements are True or False according to the text.

1. Medical triage is usually conducted by the Force Medical Officer.

2. Different health care organizations may adopt different triage classifications.

3. A 4-categrory triage system is adopted by the UN based on clinical judgement and urgency for treatment.

4. If a black tag is seen on a patient, he/she is in the most serious condition and needs to be evacuated immediately.

5. Treatment should focus on resuscitation and stabilization of casualties at the low level of medical support.

6. Evacuation of a casualty may happen withing the Mission area or out of the area.

7. Casualty evacuation to a Level 2 or 3 facility should be finished within an hour from the injury time.

8. It is the Director of MSD who decides whether evacuated patients will return to the duty station or not.

9. Once an individual is repatriated, further medical care is a national responsibility.

10. All medical units within the Mission area should prepare for mass casualty situations and disasters.

B. Directions: Answer the following questions according to your understanding of the text.

1. What is the purpose of medical triage?

2. What conditions are considered as the highest priority for treatment or evacuation in the UN operations?

3. What are the considerations in balancing the treatment capability and the availability of evacuation?

4. Who is responsible for planning and establishing medical evacuation systems?

5. What is the key criterion in determining timing and means of evacuation between levels of care?

6. Whose approval should be sought before medevac in non-emergency cases? And how about in emergencies?

7. When should medical repatriation be considered?

8. Who is responsible for the travel expenses during repatriation?

9. What should medical units do in the acute phase in face of mass casualty or disaster?

10. How to manage the dead during a mass casualty situation or a disaster?

II. Vocabulary

Directions: Choose the best word or expression from the list given for each blank. Use each word or expression only once and make proper changes when necessary.

anticipate   dictate   resuscitate   hostile

defer   mobilize   deteriorate   correspondingly

1. Drinking may make a person feel relaxed and happy, or it may make her _____, violent, or depressed.

2. After a long period, alcoholism can _____ the liver, the brain and other parts of the body.

3. Because 60-year-olds are physically in better shape now, _____, they're getting more adventurous.

4. When you _____ design decisions, you're reserving your option to change.

5. We need someone who can _____ and respond to changes in the fashion industry.

6. The meeting is an attempt to _____ nations to save children from death by disease and malnutrition.

7. The doctors managed to _____ her, but she remained in critical condition.

8. What rights does one country have to _____ the environmental standards of another?

III. Topics for Discussion

1. Please explain the 4-category triage system adopted in the UN medical treatment.

2. What elements determine the treatment and holding policy in the UN medical operations?

3. Please compare medical evacuation and medical repatriation in terms of definitions, policies and procedures.

4. What medical support should be planned in face of mass casualty and disasters at different medical levels?

<h1 align="center">Text B</h1>

<h1 align="center">The Challenges and Ethical Dilemmas of a Military Medical Officer Serving with a Peacekeeping Operation in Regard to the Medical Care of the Local Population</h1>

J. Tobin

Military medical officers are assigned to support the military personnel involved in peacekeeping operations. Their primary duty of care is to the peacekeepers. In this regard they are supported by the medical support section of the Department of Peace Keeping Operations (DPKO)[1]. The mission statement of the medical support section of the DPKO is: "[the] United Nations Support Mission is to secure the health and wellbeing of members of United Nations Peace Keeping Operations, through planning, coordination, execution, monitoring, and professional supervision of excellent medical care". Nothing is mentioned about providing medical support for the surrounding civilian population, though many peacekeeping military medical officers do this in practice. There is a requirement that they are sensitive to the social and cultural needs of the local population and are able to liaise seamlessly with the aid agencies.

Military medical officers have an ethical obligation to provide what medical aid they can to the surrounding indigenous population. In their *Regulations in Time of Armed Conflict* (the Declaration of Havana[2]), published in 1956, the World Medical Association stated: "medical ethics in time of armed conflict are identical to medical ethics in time of peace". They make no distinction between doctors serving purely in the military from other doctors working in a civilian practice. The Declaration of Havana was to function as the World Medical Association's translation of the Geneva Conventions[3] into practical guidelines for doctors. The first regulation of the Declaration of Havana states that: "The primary obligation of a physician is his professional duty; in performing his professional duty the physician's supreme guide is his conscience". The declaration also emphasizes that the key duties of physicians are focused on the relationship between the physician and the individual patient, which includes maintaining patient confidentiality, acting in the best interest of the patients, and respecting the rights of patients.

The Boston based organization, Physicians for Human Rights[4], recognized that there were unique factors that they considered were specific for peacekeeping operations. In their report, *Dual Loyalty and Human Rights*, published in 2003, they stated: "In such operations, military health professionals confront the medical needs of the civilian populations in the area of their assignment; yet they may be subject to rules and regulations preventing them from providing professional assistance to civilians". They recommended that medical personnel should resist the culture of their military colleagues and remain loyal to the ethical standards of their civilian medical colleagues.

There are natural tensions between the military medical officers and their military colleagues. In his commentary on the role of the Dutch Battalion in the fall of Srebrenica in 1995, Lt Col Vermeulen reported there were major differences of views between the leadership of the military unit and its medical staff. He failed to recognize that the unit's medical officers also had an ethical obligation to the surrounding civilian population as well as being subject to military law. The Dutch military medical officers were bound by the international code of ethics promulgated by the WMA in 1983, which states: "a physician shall give emergency care as a humanitarian duty unless he is assured that others are willing and able to give such care".

During peacekeeping operations care for the local population is normally provided by the civil local authorities, or by international aid agencies. Peacekeeping military medical officers usually become involved when these resources are either absent or inadequate. When peacekeeping military medical officers are involved in providing medical aid, they should consider the following areas: (a) medical obligations and humanitarian law, (b) the cultural and social sensitivities of civilians at a time of war, and (c) the allocation of medical resources.

Medical obligations and humanitarian law

Humanitarian provisions of the laws of war do not apply to UN peacekeeping soldiers, as they are not party to the conflict. The UN is not a state, and the UN is not a signatory to the Geneva Conventions of 1949, or to the two additional protocols of 1977. Nevertheless, the UN has adopted the position that UN troops are bound to comply with the "principles and spirit" of the conventions applicable to the conduct of military personnel. The additional protocols of 1977 stipulated that one was not permitted to distinguish between the wounded other than on medical grounds, and that medical staff were "not to be forced to refrain from acting".

In keeping with the "spirit and principles" of the Geneva Conventions, the peacekeeping military medical officer is obliged to honor Article 605, which states that "all possible measures shall be taken at all times to collect the wounded, sick, and shipwrecked and to ensure their adequate medical assistance". This was not honored during the eventual fall of Srebrenica in 1995 and the peacekeeping military medical officers were admonished in a report by the Dutch Defense Hospital Organization (KHO), for having "failed to provide adequate medical assistance to civilian casualties in a reprehensible way".

Paragraph Six of the Declaration on the Protection of Women and Children in Emergency and Armed Conflict (1974) states: "Women and children belonging to the civilian population and finding themselves in circumstances of emergency and armed conflict in the struggle for peace, self determination, national liberation and independence, or who live on / in occupied territories, shall not be deprived of shelter, medical aid or other inalienable rights".

In the Srebrenica disaster, there was conflict over "essential stock" (medical supplies) for the Dutch soldiers in case of emergency. This rationing of the "essential stock" led to the "unnecessary death" of a Bosnian woman.

It is recommended by the British Medical Association (BMA) that army doctors should thoroughly discuss ethical and potential dilemmas that may arise in advance of deployment. The BMA's recommendations were made in 2001, as a direct result of the KHO's report on the behaviour of the Dutch military medical officers at Srebrenica.

All doctors have obligations to report human rights abuses. Doctors are often among the first to witness evidence of torture, massacres or of other forms of cruel and degrading treatment. Non-governmental organizations (NGOs) and human rights organizations have argued that human rights issues are central to peacekeeping, and that human rights should be part of every peacekeeping mission and complex field operation that is launched. Physicians for Human Rights recommend that military health professionals should take steps to report violations of the Geneva Conventions.

An Australian aid worker recounted that in Rwanda, Australian peacekeepers were instructed to hold their fire when Tutsi[5] forces began to shoot into an encampment of Hutu[6] civilians at Kieho.

This ethical requirement to report abuses can possibly lead military medical officers into conflict with their own military authorities, who may be struggling to maintain a semblance of neutrality and impartiality. Impartiality is one of the key principles of UN peacekeeping. Where a peacekeeping force is perceived to have lost impartiality, "there can be no prospect of preserving the confidence and cooperation of conflicting factions". Initially, when peacekeeping was being developed, it was influenced by the superpower competition of the time. As a result, peacekeeping became an improvised alternative that was not specifically provided for in the UN Charter. Because of the politically sensitive nature of any type of third party involvement in a conflict situation, the new mechanism had to respect three basic principles: the consent of the parties to the conflict, the non-use of force, and impartiality. Since the end of the Cold War, there has been more of a focus on the humanitarian and human rights issues associated with peacekeeping.

Physicians have increasingly recognized that the promotion of health often requires the protection and promotion of human rights. Military medical officers share in this duty. Indeed they are more likely to be in situations where they will observe human rights violations first hand. Documenting human rights violations is important to establish responsibility for criminal acts, and ultimately prevent future abuses. In many ways it is akin to preventive medicine.

Social and cultural sensitivities

There is a requirement for adequate familiarization with the indigenous culture prior to setting out on the mission. For missions where multiple languages and cultures are involved, there is a requirement to communicate one's ideas, goals, and objectives to the local population, while sustaining mutual understanding and respect for each other's customs and cultural sensitivities. Local people may have expectations that are different from those of the foreign peacekeeping contingent. An example is provided by the need to assess the population's humanitarian needs. The population is aware that it is being assessed, and if there is a lack of action, this can lead to an enormous sense of frustration. A decision may have been reached by the peacekeeping force that a threshold for humanitarian intervention is higher than that which the indigenous population expects.

The peacekeeping contingent should not see itself as a factor outside the events happening around them. They should view themselves as one element in a situation, not some deus ex machina[7] immune to criticism, accountability or control.

The support of the local population is essential to the success of a peacekeeping operation. Lack of local support not only hinders the operation in the implementation of its mandate and the conduct of its daily activities, but can also pose a physical danger to the mission's personnel. Respect for the cultural traditions and social mores of the local population is essential. Providing medical services is part of the "peace building" component of the mission.

War has a destabilizing effect on the community. In the 1990s many of the wars involved regimes at war with sectors of their own society. The traditional ways for handling crises may be ineffectual, which can leave people feeling vulnerable and helpless. War tears apart the social fabric, and community structures may not be able to fill their customary role as a source of support and adaptation. It would be a mistake to view the local population in terms of victims, even though some will have developed physical and emotional problems secondary to the conflict.

A key element of modern political violence is the creation of states of terror to penetrate the entire society as a means of social control. Mozambique in the 1980s is an example: Renamo guerillas murdered around 150,000 peasants, displaced three million others, and left the social fabric of large areas in tatters. Such factors can leave the population vulnerable to exploitation, not only from the warring factions, but also from those who come to aid them.

The potential of exploitation by peacekeepers and humanitarian agencies arose in 2002. Two consultants who had been commissioned by the United Nations High Commissioner for Refugees (UNHCR)[8] and Save the Children [9](UK) reported that there was widespread sexual exploitation of refugees by humanitarian aid workers and peacekeepers in Guinea, Liberia, and Sierra Leone (UN press release: Allegations of widespread sexual exploitation in West Africa refugee camps not confirmed by United Nations investigations, 22 October 2002).

The Office of Internal Oversight Services (OIOS)[10] of the UN conducted an investigation at the request of the United Nations High Commissioner for Refugees. They found that no allegation against UN staff could be substantiated.

The OIOS identified several factors that contribute to potential exploitation of refugees, noting aspects of refugee camp life, camp structure, camp security, and aid distribution. They advised that remedial action be taken by the UNHCR and the UN Department of Peacekeeping Operations. Refugee camps have a regimenting and containing aspect to them, which places the aid agencies in a position of power in regard to the refugees. If offenders belonging to the United Nations are identified, they could be considered to be immune from the legal process of the host government under the Convention on the Privileges and Immunities of the United Nations. When this protection is used, it is expected that the officials or peacekeepers will be prosecuted by their respective home authorities. The Secretary General, or the Security Council, can waive the immunity, under the Conventions.

Though populations may have endured years of war and terror, it is unwise to assume that they are in some way rendered helpless and vulnerable. The resilience of people should not be underestimated. As Summerfield noted, even in the refugee camps in Rwanda, after the genocide of 1994, 57% of the people saw their future as being good, and 75% felt they were able to protect their families and themselves.

The allocation of medical resources

In his address to the International Peace Academy, the Secretary General of the UN, Koffi Annan, stated: "our impartial benevolence is not neutral in its effects" (UN press release: Secretary General's address to the International Peace Academy on 20 Nov 2000, SG/SM/7632, 20 November 2000).

Humanitarian assistance can be manipulated by warring factions and unscrupulous regimes for their own political purposes. Particularly in complex emergencies, humanitarian aid can fall into the hands of the warring parties. An example of this is the situation that arose in Goma, Zaire, in 1994. The refugee camps were under the strict control of the Interhamwe and the ex FAR (Forces Armees Rwandaises). This led to some of the humanitarian supplies being obtained by the genocidaires who ran the camps and launched military raids into Rwanda.

The primary responsibility for the care of a population falls upon the local authorities. It is only if they fail, or are unable to meet their humanitarian duty, that humanitarian organizations should step in to remind them of their responsibilities toward the victims, and if necessary, to take the practical measures required.

Many troop contributing countries provide humanitarian relief through their respective contingents, outside an international framework policy, or an integrated command and control center. This has the undesirable effect of making aid distribution uneven. If the mandated area of peacekeeping operations has a mixed hostile population, it can be perceived that the humanitarian and medical aid favours one population over another, as the different contingents in the operational area will have different levels of humanitarian and medical resources.

Currently, United Nations contingents are expected to bring in 90 days supply of medical consumables when entering into the Mission area. These supplies are supposed to be for their own use. To bring in medical supplies for the civilian population as well may make the operation too unwieldy and prohibitively expensive for some troop contributing countries.

Conclusion

United Nations peacekeeping military medical officers can often be faced with ethical dilemmas in regard to their duties of care toward the surrounding civilian population. They are frequently unprepared for the challenges facing them in this regard, and there is little guidance available to them. This area of medical ethics is only now being explored.

These areas of ethical dilemmas also are present for soldiers serving in national armies in times of war. The doctor may not have control of his medical supplies, but he/she does have control over his/her medical expertise. This expertise should be for the benefit of the most needy, independent of status, in a conflict zone.

(This article is excepted from "The challenges and ethical dilemmas of a military medical officer serving with a peacekeeping operation in regard to the medical care of the local population" published in *Journal of Medical Ethics,* PMID: 16199596)

Notes

1. the Department of Peace Keeping Operations (DPKO): The Department of Peace Operations is a department of the United Nations charged with the planning, preparation, management and direction of UN peacekeeping operations. Previously known as the Department for Peacekeeping Operations, it was created on 1 January 2019 as part of a restructuring of the UN's peace and security apparatus. The DPKO retains the core functions and responsibilities of its predecessor, with a greater emphasis on cohesion, integrating different resources and knowledge, and promoting human rights. 维持和平行动部

2. the Declaration of Havana: The Havana Declaration of 1960, or the First Havana Declaration, was adopted by the First National General Assembly of the people of Cuba on Sept. 2, 1960, in Havana. The declaration was the response of the people of Cuba to the American administration's attempt to isolate Cuba, Fidel Castro delivered a series of speeches designed to radicalize Latin American society. 《哈瓦那宣言》

3. the Geneva Conventions: a series of international treaties concluded in Geneva between 1864 and 1949 for the purpose of ameliorating the effects of war on soldiers and civilians. Two additional protocols to the 1949 agreement were approved in 1977. 《日内瓦公约》

4. Physicians for Human Rights: a US-based not-for-profit human rights NGO established in 1986 that uses medicine and science to document and advocate against mass atrocities and severe human rights violations around the world. PHR headquarters are in New York City, with offices in Boston and Washington, D.C. 医生促进人权组织

5. Tutsi: refers to the people who live in the densely populated African countries of Rwanda, Burundi, and in border areas of neighboring countries. They are the second largest ethnic group in Rwanda, and Burundi. 图西族

6. Hutu: a Bantu ethnic or social group native to the African Great Lakes region of Africa. They live mainly in Rwanda, Burundi and the eastern Democratic Republic of the Congo. They are traditionally a farming people and were historically dominated by the Tutsi people; the antagonism between the peoples led in 1994 to large-scale ethnic violence, especially in Rwanda. 胡图族

7. deus ex machina: (literary) an unexpected power or event that saves a situation that seems without hope, especially in a play or novel （尤指剧本或小说中）扭转乾坤之力量

8. the United Nations High Commissioner for Refugees (UNHCR): a UN agency mandated to aid and protect refugees, forcibly displaced communities, and stateless people, and to assist in their voluntary repatriation, local integration or resettlement to a third country. It was founded in 1950 and headquartered in Geneva, Switzerland, with over 17,300 staff working in 135 countries. 联合国难民事务高级专员

9. Save the Children: The Save the Children Fund, commonly known as Save the

Children, was established in the United Kingdom in 1919 to improve the lives of children through better education, health care, and economic opportunities, as well as providing emergency aid in natural disasters, war, and other conflicts. It is now a global movement made up of 29 national member organizations which works in 120 countries. 英国救助儿童会

10. the Office of Internal Oversight Services (OIOS): an independent office in the United Nations Secretariat whose mandate is to "assist the Secretary-General in fulfilling his internal oversight responsibilities in respect of the resources and staff of the Organization." Specifically, activities include internal audit, investigation, monitoring, evaluation, inspection, reporting and support services to the United Nations Secretariat. 内部监督服务司

Words and Expressions

1. liaise: *v.* (with somebody) (especially BrE.) to work closely with somebody and exchange information with them（与某人）联络，联系

2. indigenous: *adj.* belonging to the country in which they are found, rather than coming there or being brought there from another country 本土的；当地的

3. conscience: *n.* the part of your mind that tells you whether what you are doing is right or wrong 良知

4. confidentiality: *n.* a situation in which you expect somebody to keep information secret 保密性；机密性

5. be bound by: If you are bound by something such as a rule, agreement, or restriction, you are forced or required to act in a certain way. 约束

6. promulgate: *v.* to make known or public the terms of (a proposed law) 颁布；公布

7. signatory: *n.* the people, organizations, or countries that have signed an official document 签约人；签约组织；签约国

8. refrain: *v.* to keep oneself from doing, feeling, or indulging in something and especially from following a passing impulse. 忍住；克制

9. admonish: *v.* to tell someone very seriously that they have done something wrong. 告诫

10. reprehensible: *adj.* worthy of or deserving reprehension 应受斥责的；应该谴责的

11. inalienable: *adj.* incapable of being alienated, surrendered, or transferred 不能转让的；不可剥夺的

12. semblance: *n.* something that appears to exist, even though this may be a false impression 表象；外观

13. be akin to: to be similar to it in some way 与……相似

14. substantiate: *v.* to supply evidence which proves that it is true 证实

15. resilience: *n.* the ability of people or things to feel better quickly after something unpleasant, such as shock or injury 快速恢复的能力；适应力

16. genocide: *n.* the deliberate murder of a whole community or race 大屠杀

17. faction: *n.* an organized group of people within a larger group, which opposes some of the ideas of the larger group and fights for its own ideas 派系

18. unscrupulous: *adj.* prepared to act in a dishonest or immoral way to get what they want 不诚实的；不道德的

19. raid: *n.* a sudden armed attack with the aim of causing damage rather than occupying any of the enemy's land 突袭

20. unwieldy: *adj.* difficult to move or carry because it is so big or heavy 笨重的

Exercise

Critical Thinking

Dr. Tobin notes in the article that medical officers serving with their national contingents in peacekeeping operations are faced with difficult ethical decisions in regard to their obligations to the local civilian population. The medical officer has a duty to do his/her best to prevent abuse or to bring it to an end. However, at times there may be conflict with one's own military superiors. What is your opinion about the dilemma between the ethics of medical care to vulnerable civilians and fulfillment of military missions? Please state your argument and try to make it more convincing by offering evidence.

Supplementary Reading

For more information on Medical Treatment for UN Peacekeeping Operations, please go to the following websites:

1. https://cdn.peaceopstraining.org/course_promos/logistics_1/logistics_1_english.pdf

2. https://www.ipinst.org/wp-content/uploads/2017/04/IPI-Rpt-Medical-Support-Final.pdf

3. https://www.ipinst.org/wp-content/uploads/2015/03/IPI_Rpt_Health_and_Peacekeeping.pdf

Unit Four   Combat Care and Treatment

Text A
The "Top 10" Research and Development Priorities
for Battlefield Surgical Care

Matthew J. Martin

The US Military has achieved the highest casualty survival rates in its history. However, there remain multiple areas in combat trauma that present challenges to the delivery of high-quality and effective trauma care.

The organization and areas of responsibility in modern US battlefield care can roughly be grouped into three categories: (1) point of injury and prehospital care, (2) care during transport to a medical treatment facility (en-route care), and (3) forward surgical care. Although the overall goal of this system is to provide seamless care along the spectrum from injury to medical evacuation out of the combat zone, each of these areas has unique capabilities, challenges, and needs to deliver optimal care. Addressing these areas of knowledge-deficit or suboptimal capabilities has been a core focus of multiple government-funded research and development programs, such as the Combat Casualty Care Research Program (CCCRP). To optimally target and then fund research projects to address these existing "research gaps," a system for reliably identifying, characterizing, and prioritizing them must be used.

Arguably the most important organizational advance during this most recent combat experience has been the establishment of the Joint Trauma System (JTS)[1], which performs broad process and quality improvement initiatives, maintains the Department of Defense Trauma Registry (DODTR)[2], and supports the CCCRP in helping to identify key research and development priorities. As a critical component of these activities, the JTS has established three committees with areas of focus and responsibility that correspond to the three phases of care outlined above (pre-hospital, en-route care, and forward surgical care). The earliest and arguably most successful of these has been the Committee on Tactical Combat Casualty Care (CoTCCC). The work of this committee led to major improvements in the quality and standardization of battlefield trauma care, and has been widely recognized as a key contributor to the historically low case fatality rates seen during the past 15 years of combat operations. An additional landmark work-product of the CoTCCC was the identification and publication of a list of prioritized gaps in need of focused research and development. Since publication, this "Top 10" list has been an invaluable resource for researchers and research administrators in both the civilian and military communities. However, this effort was primarily focused on interventions and care-related gaps at the point-of-injury and prehospital phases, and did not address some of the different issues or specific challenges in subsequent phases of care. Based on the major successes achieved by the CoTCCC, the JTS established two additional committees: the Committee on En-Route Casualty Care (CoERCC) that focuses on care during the medical transport and evacuation phases, and the Committee on Surgical Combat Casualty Care (CoSCCC) that focuses on care at forward medical treatment facilities (MTFs) with surgical capabilities (Role 2 or 3 care).

A list of critical "focus areas" was developed by the Committee on Surgical Combat Casualty Care (CoSCCC). The top five focus areas were Personnel/Staffing, Resuscitation and Hemorrhage Management, Pain/Sedation/Anxiety Management, Operative Interventions, and Initial Evaluation. The "Top 10" specific research topics were identified (actual total of 11 topics as a result of a tie score for no. 10) and are listed along with their corresponding focus area in Table 4-1. The "Top 10" research priorities were all from three focus areas, including four in Personnel/Staffing, four in Resuscitation/Hemorrhage Management, and three in Operative Interventions.

This is the first objective ranking of research priorities for combat trauma care. This data will help guide Department of Defense research programs and new areas for prioritized funding of both military and civilian researchers.

Table 4-1   The "Top 10" Research Priorities for Forward Surgical Care

Research Topic	Focus Area	Score (Mean)
1. Assessment of actual capabilities and potential benefit versus harm associated with the use of small "austere surgical teams" versus standard-sized forward surgical teams	Personnel/Staffing	8.46
2. Optimization of blood products and their storage for transfusion	Resuscitation and Initial Hemorrhage Management	8.22
3. Optimal number, mix, and training of personnel for variety of missions/scenarios	Personnel/Staffing	8.17
4. Non-operative interventions for non-compressible truncal hemorrhage	Resuscitation and Initial Hemorrhage Management	8.13
5. Damage control interventions for exsanguinating abdominal hemorrhage	Operative interventions	7.92
6. Effect of operating room team skillset composition on surgical outcomes	Operative interventions	7.77
7. Outcomes analysis and comparisons based on unit size and composition	Personnel/Staffing	7.77
8. Damage control interventions for major vascular injuries	Operative interventions	7.75
9. Analysis of operative case-loads and mix, and skills required to determine staffing needs	Personnel/Staffing	7.73
10 A. REBOA*—improving access routes/methods, guiding device placement, monitoring effectiveness	Resuscitation and Initial Hemorrhage Management	7.72
10B. Factor concentrates and alternative products for hemostatic resuscitation	Resuscitation and Initial Hemorrhage Management	7.72

* REBOA, resuscitative endovascular balloon occlusion of the aorta.

Personnel and Staffing (Number, Mix, Capabilities)

Surprisingly to the authors, the top identified research priority and the highest priority focus area were both related to the non-clinical topic of staffing and capabilities for forward surgical elements. In fact, four of the top 10 priorities were related to this focus area, and we believe represents the major concerns and lack of data associated with recent changes and deviations from standard combat medical support doctrine. Chief among these has been the increasing use of smaller and less well-equipped teams to provide forward surgical care, and supporting combat operations in a role that had traditionally been handled by either complete or split Role 2 elements such as the Army Forward Surgical Team. These teams now come in a variety of sizes and configurations, generally consist of less than 10 personnel, and are broadly identified now as "austere surgical teams." They also vary widely in the amount and depth of predeployment team training they complete, their equipment and supply chain, and the types of operations they are supporting. Among the greatest concerns with the use of these teams is the near complete lack of objective data to assess their effectiveness, strengths and limitations, and patient outcomes. We believe that improved and mandatory data collection and analyses related to these teams should be a top priority, and that they should be used with caution and careful oversight to ensure that acceptable care and outcomes are being achieved. In addition to the identified priority of research regarding these teams, the CoSCCC is also currently developing a new JTS Clinical Practice Guideline focused on austere surgical teams.

Additional research priorities in the Top 10 under this focus area were related to identifying optimal size, numbers, and personnel mix among doctrinal Role 2 and 3 units, and their relationship to outcomes in a variety of operational settings. In addition to the use of austere surgical teams, there have been major changes and variability in the deployment of standard Role 2 and 3 units, as well as changes to the personnel and specialty mix. Both Role 2 and 3 facilities have frequently been split into two or more smaller elements, with each expected to function as an independent MTF in support of forward operations. There have also been significant changes in terms of the staffing doctrine for Role 2 teams, with the most recent change being the addition of Emergency Medicine providers and reduction in the number of surgeons. The ultimate effect (if any) of these changes has not been well studied, and should be another top research priority for the DOD. Finally, there is a need for research and analyses to identify the optimal mix of operative team personnel, specialties, training, and readiness status to achieve optimal outcomes in the demanding combat environment. However, this area is an excellent illustrative example of a multifaceted problem that will require solutions that go beyond simple medical research or research funding, and that will require input and changes related to staffing and training doctrines, procurement and equipping, medical planning and layout, and robust informatics capture and analysis.

Resuscitation and Hemorrhage Management

The identification of this focus area related to the management and resuscitation of the bleeding combat trauma patient as a top priority is not surprising and is supported by the consistent finding of hemorrhage being the most common cause of preventable battlefield deaths. This also represents a clear overlap with the priorities identified by the CoTCCC and those in development by the CoERCC. Although the majority of deaths and research focus on early hemorrhage control have been in the pre-hospital environment, several analyses of in-hospital deaths have emphasized that hemorrhage control remains among the most common causes of preventable mortality and morbidity after arrival at an MTF. This represents an area that has clearly seen great progress through the use of rapid and gap-driven research programs, and that has resulted in major advances in hemorrhage control techniques and devices, training programs, and strategies for resuscitation.

Several areas of much-needed research in this focus area were identified as top priorities in this analysis. With the rise of blood products as the preferred initial resuscitative fluid for bleeding combat trauma victims, there is a great need to study methods to optimize blood products for use in the austere environment, to prolong and simplify the storage requirements, and to minimize the associated complications and adverse effects that can occur with transfusion. In addition to standard blood products, there is a renewed interest in pharmacologic adjuncts (such as tranexamic acid) and in factor concentrate products as potentially more effective and efficient options for resuscitation and correction of coagulopathy. There is also a clear need for effective nonoperative interventions for hemorrhage control, and particularly for truncal hemorrhage, that can serve as a bridge to facilitate movement to the operating room. There is currently great interest in resuscitative endovascular balloon occlusion of the aorta (REBOA) as a viable option for this indication, although much additional research is needed to clarify the indications, techniques, required training, and methods to minimize the ischemia-reperfusion[3] caused by prolonged REBOA. Finally, given the limitations in availability and usability of advanced invasive monitoring in the forward environment, another top priority is the development and testing of new non-invasive hemodynamic monitoring systems to aid in the early identification of patients with major bleeding or early shock and to guide resuscitation.

Operative Interventions

As the defining characteristic of a Role 2 or higher facility is the presence of a surgeon and a surgical team capable of performing major operative interventions, it is not surprising that this focus area would be among the top-ranked priorities. This is an area that distinguishes this analysis from previous ones that have focused on issues relevant to the environment outside of a fixed MTF. This is also an area that somewhat overlaps with other identified priorities, such as resuscitation of the bleeding patient, and optimal staffing and capabilities to provide effective surgical intervention. New research efforts in this focus area must consider not only the general issues related to major trauma surgery for combat injuries but also the wide variability in surgical capabilities and primary missions of different types of deployed units. For example, the core mission of a deployed Role 2 facility is typically limited to performing major damage-control surgery and then transfer to the next echelon of care. This is contrasted to the mission of a standard Role 3 facility, where the more robust capabilities and holding capacity allow for more definitive surgical care and complex reconstructions.

In addition to the already listed research priorities around staffing and capabilities mix, the development of improved techniques and adjuncts for major damage control surgery are needed and should be a high priority. New devices or techniques that facilitate and expand the ability of the surgeon to achieve control of hemorrhage and gastrointestinal spillage may be associated with improved outcomes, and also with an improved ability to conserve scarce resources such as blood products and operating room time. New developments for the management of major vascular injuries were also identified among the top 10 priorities, as these injuries are frequently among the most challenging and high risk for adverse outcomes. This is a particularly important priority given the widely identified problem of decreasing exposure to open vascular surgery and vascular trauma cases among graduating surgical residents, which results in less experience and comfort with the definitive management of these injuries on the battlefield. Adjuncts to assist in obtaining rapid hemorrhage control, re-establishing arterial flow, and performing temporary or definitive reconstruction (such as shunts, stents, sutureless anastomoses, etc.) will require further focused research and development programs.

Conclusions

This work represents the initial development and analysis of a rank-ordered list of research gaps and priorities to inform combat casualty care research related to the delivery of battlefield surgical care at the Role 2 and 3 levels. This includes a list of the "Top 10" research priorities, all of which came from one of three high priority focus areas related to personnel and staffing, resuscitation and hemorrhage control, and major operative interventions. Despite including responses from a highly heterogeneous group of experts, we found an extremely high degree of agreement and inter-rater correlation for the rankings and prioritization process. In addition to pure scientific research aligned with these priorities, solutions to the challenges of forward surgical care will require changes in military doctrine, training, education, logistics, personnel, facilities, and organizational structure that are now a priority focus of the JTS and other elements of the DOD.

(This article is excerpted from "The 'Top 10' research and development priorities for battlefield surgical care: Results from the Committee on Surgical Combat Casualty Care research gap analysis" published in *Journal of Trauma Acute Care Surgery*, PMID: 31246901)

Notes

1. Joint Trauma System (JTS): the DOD authority responsible for trauma system development, trauma system performance improvement, trauma data collection, and trauma registry translational research 联合创伤系统

2. Department of Defense (DOD): America's largest government agency. The Defense Department has 11 combatant commands, each with a geographic or functional mission that provides command and control of military forces in peace and war. The Army, Marine Corps, Navy, Air Force, Space Force and Coast Guard are the armed forces of the United States. 美国国防部

3. ischemia-reperfusion: tissue ischemia with inadequate oxygen supply followed by successful reperfusion initiates a wide and complex array of inflammatory responses that may both aggravate local injury as well as induce impairment of remote organ function 缺血再灌注

Words and Expressions

1. spectrum: *n.* any range or scale, as of capabilities, emotions, or moods 范围

2. multifaceted: *adj.* having many different aspects to be considered 多方面的；多层面的

3. austere: *adj.* severely simple or plain 朴素的，简朴的

4. truncal: *adj.* relating to the trunk of the body or to any arterial or nerve trunk, etc. 躯干的

5. civilian: *n./adj.* a person who is not an active member of the military, the police, or a belligerent group in a conflict 平民（的）

6. doctrine: *n.* a rule or principle of law, especially when established by precedent 原则

7. configuration: *n.* an arrangement of the parts of something or a group of things; the form or shape that this arrangement produces 布局；结构；配置

8. mandatory: *adj.* required by law or rule 强制的；命令的

9. demanding: *adj.* needing a lot of skill, patience, effort, etc. 要求高的；需要高技能（或耐性等）的；费力的

Medical Vocabulary

hemorrhage: 出血

exsanguinate: 失血

transfusion: 输血

coagulopathy: 凝血障碍

resuscitation: 复苏

occlusion: 梗塞

indication: 适应症

fatality rate: 病死率

endovascular: 血管内的

aorta: 主动脉

pharmacologic: 药理学的

tranexamic acid: 氨甲环酸；凝血酸

hemodynamic: 血液动力学的

gastrointestinal: 胃肠的

spillage: 溢液；溢出物

shunt: 分流术

stent: 支架术

sutureless anastomoses: 无缝线吻合术

Exercises

I. Reading Comprehension

A. Directions: Decide whether the following statements are True or False according to the text.

1. The US Military has achieved the highest casualty survival rates in its history.

2. The Committee on En-Route Casualty Care (CoERCC) focuses on care at forward medical treatment facilities (MTFs) with surgical capabilities.

3. The top 10 research priorities were all from three focus areas.

4. Three of the top 10 priorities were related to the focus area of Personnel and Staffing.

5. "Austere surgical teams" now come in a variety of sizes and configurations, generally composed of more than 10 personnel.

6. There has been increasing use of smaller and less well-equipped teams to provide forward surgical care.

7. It has been consistently found that hemorrhage is the most common cause of preventable battlefield deaths.

8. The Joint Trauma System (JTS) supports the CCCRP in helping to identify key research and development priorities.

B. Directions: Answer the following questions according to your understanding of the text.

1. How many categories can the areas of responsibility in modern US battlefield care be grouped into?

2. What are the three committees established by the JTS?

3. Where is a renewed interest for resuscitation and correction of coagulopathy?

4. What is one of the greatest concerns with the use of "austere surgical teams"?

5. What needs to be done immediately with the rise of blood products as the preferred initial resuscitative fluid for bleeding combat trauma victims?

6. What can serve as a bridge to facilitate movement to the operating room?

7. What new research efforts must be considered in the focus area of Operative Interventions?

8. What is the consequence of decreasing exposure to open vascular surgery and vascular trauma cases among graduating surgical residents?

II. Vocabulary

Directions: Choose the best word or expression from the list given for each blank. Use each word or expression only once and make proper changes when necessary.

demanding   civilian   mandatory   doctrine

austere   multifaceted   spectrum   configuration

1. Politicians across the political _____ have denounced the act.

2. The life of the troops was still comparatively _____.

3. He tried to return to work, but found he could no longer cope with his _____ job.

4. Fall prevention strategies should be comprehensive and _____.

5. The safety of _____ caught up in the fighting must be guaranteed.

6. Things that might have been optional in the past for job seekers are now _____.

7. Prices range from $119 to $199, depending on the particular _____.

8. Like communism, the _____ of socialism demands state ownership and equal distribution of wealth.

III. Topics for Discussion

1. What do you think are the top three priorities among the "Top 10" research and development priorities for battlefield surgical care? Please have a discussion with your classmates.

2. Please collect the latest news about battlefield surgical care in China and share it with your classmates.

Text B

A Machine Learning-Based Model to Predict Acute Traumatic Coagulopathy in Trauma Patients upon Emergency Hospitalization

Tanshi Li

Introduction

Annually, traumatic injury leads to more than 5 million deaths worldwide, comprising 10% of global mortality, and trauma care is thus a huge burden on medical resources and health services. Uncontrolled hemorrhage is associated with 40% of traumatic deaths, and among such cases, 60% of hemorrhagic deaths occur within 3 hours of admission and a total of 94% occur within 24 hours. A variety of factors contribute to massive bleeding, yet acute traumatic coagulopathy (ATC) is widely considered to be a leading cause, affecting up to 30% of severely injured patients; indeed, ATC is understood to predict up to 4-fold increases in bleeding-related mortality.

Acute traumatic coagulopathy is an endogenous coagulopathy multifactorial with many mechanisms, including tissue damage, shock, hemodilution, hypothermia, acidemia, inflammation, and hypoperfusion, and early detection and intervention of ATC is known to significantly reduce mortality and to ameliorate the outcomes of trauma patients. Therefore, it is of great importance to develop prediction models that can alert clinicians to potential ATC cases when trauma patients arrive at the emergency department (ED). Ideally, such models would have the following characteristics: (1) Simplicity: The model needs to be based on data that are easily accessible upon admission to the ED. (2) Universality: Indicators for building models can be widely applied to medical institutions around the world. (3) Timeliness: Observed indicators can be obtained quickly, helping doctors get prediction results rapidly and enabling them to take model-guided interventions in time.

Several previous studies have reported the development of predictive models for ATC, including, for example, the Prediction of Acute Coagulopathy of Trauma (PACT) score. The PACT score is primarily based on prehospital treatment data including age, injury mechanism, prehospital Shock Index, Glasgow Coma Score[1] values, prehospital cardiopulmonary resuscitation, and endotracheal intubation. However, due to the distinct prehospital practice patterns and variation in the experience and technical backgrounds of ambulance crew in different countries, these subjective variables are ultimately limited in clinical application. In short, there is a great opportunity to use objective clinical features assessed upon admission to the ED to develop more powerful predictive models for ACT.

To date, the diagnosis of ATC has been based on conventional coagulation indicators such as activated partial thromboplastin time, prothrombin time, and international normalized ratio (INR)[2], among others, and these typically require a minimum of 1 to 2 hours of processing time after admission to the ED. This time lag can result in the loss of therapeutic windows for treating ATC. Notably, a previous study with ATC cases showed that an INR >1.5 during admission to the ED is associated with multiple adverse prognoses. So, it is of vital importance to develop a prediction model that can identify ATC rapidly because it could inform ancillary resource management and clinical decision support to help save the lives of trauma patients.

Here, we used machine learning methods (eg, random forest algorithm) to develop and validate a prediction model for ATC that is based on objective indicators which are already routinely obtained as patients are admitted to the hospital. Our study also developed a predictive model based on a more traditional logistic regression method, enabling us to rigorously compare the performance of the 2 models.

Methods and Results

Using the critical care Emergency Rescue Database and further collected data in ED, a total of 1,385 patients were analyzed and cases with initial international normalized ratio (INR) values>1.5 upon admission to the ED met the defined diagnostic criteria for ATC; nontraumatic conditions with potentially disordered coagulation systems were excluded. A total of 818 individuals were collected from Emergency Rescue Database as derivation cohorts, who were then split 7:3 into training and test data sets. A Pearson correlation matrix was used to initially identify likely key clinical features associated with ATC, and analysis of data distributions was undertaken prior to the selection of suitable modeling tools. Both machine learning (random forest) and traditional logistic regression were deployed for prediction modeling of ATC. After the model was established, another 587 patients were collected in the ED as validation cohorts. The ATC prediction models incorporated red blood cell count, Shock Index, base excess, lactate, diastolic blood pressure, and potential of hydrogen. Of 818 trauma patients screened from the database, 747 (91.3%) patients did not present ATC (INR 1.5) and 71 (8.7%) patients had ATC (INR > 1.5) upon admission to the ED. Compared to the logistic regression model, the model based on the random forest algorithm showed better accuracy (94.0%, 95% confidence interval [CI]: 0.922-0.954 to 93.5%, 95% CI: 0.916-0.95), precision (93.3%, 95% CI: 0.914-0.948 to 93.1%, 95% CI: 0.912-0.946), F1 score (93.4%, 95% CI: 0.915-0.949 to 92%, 95% CI: 0.9-0.937), and recall score (94.0%, 95% CI: 0.922- 0.954 to 93.5%, 95% CI: 0.916-0.95) but yielded a lower area under the receiver operating characteristic curve (AU-ROC) (0.810, 95% CI: 0.673-0.918 to 0.849, 95% CI: 0.732-0.944) for predicting ATC in trauma patients.

Discussion

In this study, by establishing 2 predictive models for ATC, we screened for admission indicators that are informative for the onset of ATC. With our newly developed models—both of which incorporated only 6 objective and readily obtainable indicators that are already universally available during admission to the ED—we can very confidently predict patients at risk for ATC (random forest: accuracy 94%, precision 93.3%, recall 94%, and F1 score 93.4% vs logistic regression: accuracy 93.5%, precision 93.1%, recall 93.5%, and F1 score 92%). Preliminary inferential statistical and correlation-based analyses suggested that the most informative clinical features for ATC were likely RBC, SI, BE, Lac, DBP, and PH; findings conform with other studies.

It is important to note that both models performed very well in both test and validation samples. The discrepancy between the 2 modeling strategies is that the random forest model is better in terms of accuracy, precision, F1 score, and recall scores, while the logistic regression model offers superior predicted performance in AU-ROC. Considering that a lower rate of missed diagnosis is preferred in a medical model, the logistic model may provide more information in this given topic. Furthermore, there are many reports in literature which highlight that machine learning-based models can often outperform logistic regression models for predicting various medical outcomes, yet our study emphasizes that traditional regression-based models also often perform well. It may be because our study cohort is not large enough to show critical difference in every performance metric. Further study could be done if possible. Ultimately, our comparison of the performance of the 2 models suggests that clinical computer-aided workflows should probably combine a variety of models to capitalize on their individual strengths while overcoming any particular limitations.

Potentially pathogenic roles of RBCs in coagulopathy have been little explored until recently, yet there are now multiple studies that propose multiple functions for RBCs in hemostasis and in thrombosis in trauma patients. The hemorheological effects of RBCs can be an essential prothrombotic factor because impaired blood flow is a known pathophysiological mechanism of thrombosis. It is also known that many bleeding disorders can be treated by increasing the RBC count, regardless of the platelet level. Furthermore, RBC count is interconnected with clot contraction, fibrinolysis, and endothelium homeostasis. Our random forest model ranked RBC first in terms of feature importance, a finding which affirms previously reported findings.

Shock Index and DBP are sensitive indices of shock. Corresponding to our observation, hemorrhagic shock (HS) has been widely illustrated to be significantly correlated with the occurrence of ATC in both clinical and animal experiments. Shock Index was interpreted to be a favorable predictor of massive hemorrhage in both prehospital and ED settings, when $SI \geqslant 0.9$ postinjury can recognize patients with critical bleeding. As a primary indicator of hemodynamic monitoring, DBP may be predictive for patient mortality in cardiogenic shock and/or septic shock. For HS, the HR undergoes a compensatory increase due to hypovolemia that leads to a short diastolic phase and results in the elevation of DBP. Furthermore, ATC is associated with metabolic acidosis that originates from systemic hypoperfusion as a result of hypovolemia. As excellent indicators of hypoperfusion, BE, Lac, and PH predict higher incidence of shock-related complications such as acute respiratory distress syndrome, multi-organ failure, and the need for transfusion.

As with past prediction models like PACT score, we intended to incorporate risk stratification into our model, so we selected patients with severe injuries with triage target reported as "trauma" and narrowed down to patients who were assigned to a critical rescue room. In contrast to previous models, our model is based on the routinely obtained data that are taken during admission to the ED, rather than data acquired in a prehospital stage. On the one hand, this means our model inherently lags behind in prediction window compared to the PACT score. On the other hand, however, given that we applied objective indicators that showed strong linear relationships with the occurrence of ATC, we anticipated that our model would be extremely helpful in the ED setting, especially as computer-aided prediction and triage technologies become more common. Our study has several limitations. First, we have used admission INR>1.5 to define ATC, a value that has been well verified in both civil and military settings. However, this selected value cannot fully account for ATC pathogenesis. Multiple studies have suggested that viscoelastic tests could be effective supplements for the detection of ATC, and these have been increasingly applied in trauma situations; they provide rapid information about the underlying mechanism of ATC and allow clinicians to focus on particular aspects of clotting, facilitating targeted coagulation supervision and intervention(s) in accordance with the particular needs of a given individual. Unfortunately, the Emergency Rescue Database had relatively little information from viscoelastic test for subjects. As such tests become increasingly common, there should be adequate data to conduct follow-on analyses from our modeling work which will likely add yet better predictive performance for ATC. Second, the injury severity score (ISS) has been independently associated with increased coagulopathy, yet in practice—because of the need for staff training as well as enormous workloads and ED urgency—it is difficult to routinely calculate ISS. We did anticipate this in our study design and had intended to enroll the triage level as a potential proxy indicator for severity instead of ISS. However, our data analysis revealed that the triage level did not show an obvious correlation or importance for ATC. Perhaps triage modes could be optimized in the future to better characterize the severity of trauma. Third, our single-center study will obviously need external validation with data from other trauma centers to enhance its application.

Conclusion

We developed a prediction model based on objective, rapidly accessible data that can powerfully predict which trauma patients are at risk for ATC upon admission to the ED. An important purpose of our study is that routinely acquired objective clinical features offer a rich source of predictive power as more and more computer-aided workflows are incorporated into modern medicine. Moreover, we ultimately found that a machine learning algorithm did offer certain benefits as we developed predictive models, but our impressive predictive power from a more traditional logistic regression model also highlighted the fact that computer-aided clinical guidance tools can profit from both emerging and traditional methods from computer science and biostatistics.

(This article is excepted from "A Machine Learning-Based Model to Predict Acute Traumatic Coagulopathy in Trauma Patients Upon Emergency Hospitalization" published in *Clinical and Applied Thrombosis/Hemostasis*, PMID: 31908189)

Notes

1. Glasgow Coma Scale: (assessment of coma and impaired consciousness) The Scale was described in 1974 by Graham Teasdale and Bryan Jennett as a way to communicate about the level of consciousness of patients with an acute brain injury. The findings using the scale guide initial decision making and monitor trends in responsiveness that are important in signaling the need for new actions. 格拉斯哥昏迷指数

2. international normalized ratio (INR): International normalized ratio (INR) is the preferred test of choice for patients taking vitamin K antagonists (VKA). It can also be used to assess the risk of bleeding or the coagulation status of the patients. 国际标准化比值

Words and Expressions

1. endogenous: *adj.* (of a disease or symptom) having no obvious cause 内源性的；内生的

2. ameliorate: *v.* to make or become better; to improve 改善；减轻（痛苦等）

3. ancillary: *adj.* providing necessary support to the main work or activities of an organization 辅助的；补充的

4. discrepancy: *n.* a difference between two or more things that should be the same 差异

5. outperform: *v.* to achieve better results than somebody or something 超过，胜过

6. onset: *n.* the beginning of something, especially something unpleasant 开端，发生

Medical Vocabulary

hemodilution: 血液稀释

hypothermia: 体温过低

acidemia: 酸血症

hypoperfusion: 灌注不足；低灌注

endotracheal: 气管内的

intubation: 插管；插管法

prothrombin: 凝血酶原

thromboplastin: 促凝血酶原激酶

lactate: 乳酸

hemostasis: 止血

hemorheological: 血液流变学的

fibrinolysis: 纤维蛋白溶解

endothelium: 内皮

cardiogenic shock: 心源性休克

septic shock: 感染性休克

hypovolemia: 血容量过低

triage: 伤员检伤分类

platelet: 血小板

viscoelastic tests: 黏弹性检测

Exercise

Critical Thinking

According to this study, routinely acquired objective clinical features offer predictive power as more computer-aided workflows are incorporated into modern medicine. Have you adopted this approach in your work? If so, please share your relevant experience with your partner.

Supplementary Reading

For more information on Combat Care and Treatment, please go to the following websites:

1. https://jmvh.org/article/glimpses-of-future-battlefield-medicine-the-proliferation-of-robotic-surgeons-and-unmanned-vehicles-and-technologies/

2. https://www.battlefieldsurgeon.com/surgical-cases

3. https://journals.lww.com/jtrauma/Fulltext/1997/08000/Surgical_Lessons_Learned_on_the_Battlefield.1.aspx

Unit Five   Wound Care and Pain Relief

Text A
The Future of Wound Care

Mary Bates

Wounds, especially chronic wounds, represent a significant clinical, social, and economic challenge. A recent retrospective analysis of Medicare beneficiaries in the United States identified that about 8.2 million people had at least one type of wound, with surgical wounds and diabetic ulcers among the most common and expensive to treat. The study also found that Medicare expenditures related to wound care are far greater than previously recognized; estimates for acute and chronic wound treatments ranged from US\$28.1 billion to \$96.8 billion.

But even with the annual wound care products market expected to reach \$15-\$22 billion by 2024, many aspects of wound care have remained unchanged for decades. Now, teams of clinicians and engineers are working on new technologies that have the potential to transform wound care, making the process smarter, faster, and more efficient.

Innovative and safe treatment

Much of the research of Jeffrey Catchmark, a professor of agricultural and biological engineering at Pennsylvania State University, is focused on developing naturally derived biomaterials to reduce the world's reliance on plastics. In an attempt to come up with a Styrofoam replacement, he combined an anionic starch with a cationic chitosan (a sugar obtained from the outer skeleton of shellfish) to make a stable, insoluble foam.

Catchmark's material caught the interest of Scott Armen, chief of the division of trauma, acute care, and critical care surgery at Penn State Health Milton S. Hershey Medical Center and a colonel in the US Army Reserve[1]. He saw its potential in wound care. Together, Armen and Catchmark developed the material into a biofoam that could be placed within traumatic wounds to stop bleeding and stabilize patients.

The material starts off as more of a conventional foam, absorbing blood and body fluids and expanding to put pressure on the wound. As healing progresses, it transforms into a gel that aids in wound healing by keeping the area hydrated. In addition, the biofoam has several appealing attributes. Its ingredients are bioabsorbable and safe for long-term use. Chitosan appears to promote clotting to help stop bleeding. It is also flexible and durable, able to be molded to fit inside wounds. "There's just no other product out there that does all these things in this way," says Catchmark.

Catchmark and Armen hope to produce a to-go pack of the foam that could be easily carried and used in the field by emergency responders and military medics[2].

"This material could ultimately become a common wound care material for almost any application: traumatic wounds, surgical wounds, or everyday wounds," says Catchmark.

"It could really impact lives, all the way from soldiers on the battlefield to patients in hospitals or even home care."

On-demand, smart solution

While on a sabbatical at Harvard Medical School, Sameer Sonkusale learned that wound care was a top concern of the doctors and clinicians he met. "We've been using the same old bandages to treat wounds and the outcome hasn't improved," says Sonkusale, a professor of electrical and computer engineering at Tufts University. That observation inspired Sonkusale, along with collaborators from Harvard and Purdue University, to develop a way to monitor wound healing in real time and deliver treatments on demand.

The result is a prototype for a smart bandage. Demonstrated effective at improving healing in diabetic mice, it can actively monitor different wound biomarkers and deliver appropriate drug doses with little to no intervention needed. Sonkusale says the emergence of flexible electronics made it possible to design a smart material that is also flexible and thin enough to serve as a bandage. The prototype bandages contain heating elements and heat-responsive drug carriers capable of delivering tailored doses of antibiotics or painkillers in response to embedded pH and temperature sensors, which track infection and inflammation. By providing real-time data on how wounds are healing and delivering medicine when necessary, smart bandages like these could save time and money for patients and doctors.

"It's a problem when wounds become infected and then require more intensive treatment," says Sonkusale. "What we tried to do with this bandage is create a closed-loop system that monitors the sensors and then delivers the drug on demand."

Although this particular prototype was equipped with pH and temperature sensors and antibiotic drug delivery, Sonkusale imagines a wide range of potential applications. The type of sensors embedded in the bandage and the treatments delivered could be individualized to monitor different healing markers and treat different conditions.

Clinical trials are still needed, but Sonkusale sees a lot of opportunities for improvement to the smart bandage going forward.

"We made versions of the bandages with some features to show we can do this," he says. "But as a platform, our smart bandage is widely applicable to any kind of wound, including burns, infections, and diabetic wounds."

Remote, data-driven management

Chronic and nonhealing wounds, such as diabetic ulcers, affect millions of Americans.

One recent study showed nearly 15% of Medicare beneficiaries require treatment for at least one type of chronic wound or infection. Responding to this need, a team from the University of Nebraska-Lincoln, Harvard Medical School, and the Massachusetts Institute of Technology designed a smart bandage that can precisely deliver different medications to hard-to-treat wounds.

"This bandage combined two advancements," says Ali Tamayol, one of the device's inventors who is now at the department of biomedical engineering at the University of Connecticut. "One is mode of drug delivery and the second is in precision of drug delivery." This smart bandage is equipped with miniature needles that are able to penetrate into deeper layers of the wound, delivering drugs intradermally with minimal pain and inflammation. The needles are controlled wirelessly, allowing treatments to be programmed by care providers from afar.

In a pilot study, diabetic mice treated with the smart bandage showed signs of complete healing and lack of scar formation. The method improved the rate and quality of wound healing compared to topical administration of drugs.

Tamayol says it was important for him and his collaborators to listen to care providers and patients to understand opportunities for improvement. A top concern of patients was minimizing the need for visiting care providers so often. Care providers were interested in measures that could inform them about the conditions of the wound environment. Tamayol believes this smart bandage could do both.

Tamayol says that some of the components of the smart bandage could be altered to fit the needs of different types of wounds. While he is excited by the bandage's potential, he also acknowledges the challenges of bringing such a product onto the market soon.

"There are a lot of advancements put forward in the engineering world but getting them into clinical practice is not always feasible," says Tamayol. "The reality might be that simplified versions of some of these technologies can be incorporated into clinical practice initially and then, slowly, more complexity could be added."

Leveraging natural movement

Xudong Wang, a professor of materials science and engineering at the University of Wisconsin-Madison, has been working on generating energy from the human body for over ten years, developing wearable devices for converting body motions, such as muscle stretching, into electricity. He's recently turned his attention to the role electrical pulses play in biological processes, with an eye toward medical applications.

"Skin wounds actually use the internal electrical field on the wounded area to help with cell proliferation," says Wang. "This is how we came up with our hypothesis that we can use this body-generated electricity to stimulate wound healing and facilitate recovery."

Wang and his colleagues developed a bandage that speeds up healing by harnessing the body's own energy. The bandage uses body movements to generate gentle electrical pulses at the site of an injury, encouraging wound healing. It consists of nanogenerators that convert movements, such as ones caused by breathing, into electrical pulses. The nanogenerators are linked to a band worn around the patient's (or lab animal's) torso. The expansion and contraction of the wearer's ribcage during breathing powers the nanogenerators, which then deliver low-intensity electric pulses to the wounded area.

In laboratory tests, rats whose wounds were treated with the electric bandage healed in three days, compared to a normal two-week healing process. The results are encouraging, but Wang says further tests are needed before the technology moves into human trials. He is currently collaborating with Angela Gibson, a trauma and burn surgeon at the University of Wisconsin, to test the bandages on pigs, whose skin is more similar to that of humans, and human skin cells in the lab.

"We have tested this on acute wounds, which provide a good example for us to study how the cells are responding, but eventually we want to apply this to more serious and challenging wounds, such as chronic wounds and burns," says Wang. "Burn wounds can cover a large area and often leave scars. Electric fields are directional and this can help cells align and therefore minimize scar formation."

Wang believes the technology, which is streamlined and inexpensive, could be put to many different therapeutic uses beyond wound care. He's also demonstrated the power of his nanogenerators to encourage the growth of hair follicles and stimulate the vagus nerve near the stomach as a way to limit food intake and control obesity.

Notes

1. US Army Reserve: a reserve force of the United States Army. Together, the Army Reserve and the Army National Guard constitute the Army element of the reserve components of the United States Armed Forces. 美国陆军预备役部队

2. medic: a medical practitioner in the armed forces; military medic 军医

Words and Expressions

1. chronic: *adj.* (especially of a disease) lasting for a long time; difficult to cure or get rid of 慢性的，难以治愈（或根除）的

2. acute: *adj.* an acute illness is one that has quickly become severe and dangerous（疾病）急性的

3. range: *v.* to vary between two particular amounts, sizes, etc., including others between them（在一定的范围内）变化，变动

4. derive: *v.* to obtain a substance from something（从……中）提取

5. insoluble: *adj.* (of a substance) that does not dissolve in a liquid 不能溶解的；不溶的

6. attribute: *n.* a quality or feature of somebody/something 属性，性质，特征

7. inspire: *v.* to give somebody the idea for something, especially something artistic or that shows imagination　赋予灵感，引起联想，启发思考

8. prototype: *n.* (for/of something) the first design of something from which other forms are copied or developed　原型，雏形，最初形态

9. tailored: *adj.* made for a particular person or purpose　特制的，专门的

10. embed: *v.* to fix something firmly into a substance or solid object　把……牢牢地嵌入（或插入、埋入）

11. individualize: *v.* to make something different to suit the needs of a particular person, place, etc.　使个性化，使因人（或因地等）而异

12. miniature: *adj.* [only before noun] very small; much smaller than usual　很小的，微型的，小型的

13. penetrate: *v.* to go into or through something　穿过，进入

14. streamline: *v.* to streamline an organization or process means to make it more efficient by removing unnecessary parts of it　提高……效率

15. proliferation: *n.* the sudden increase in the number or amount of something; a large number of a particular thing　激增，涌现，增殖

16. harness: *v.* to control and use the force or strength of something to produce power or to achieve something　控制，利用（以产生能量等）

Medical Vocabulary

diabetic ulcer: 糖尿病溃疡

Styrofoam: 泡沫聚苯乙烯

anionic starch: 阴离子淀粉

cationic chitosan: 阳离子壳聚糖

intradermally: 皮内地

torso: 躯干

ribcage: 胸腔

hair follicle: 毛囊

vagus nerve: 迷走神经，交感神经

Exercises

I. Reading Comprehension

A. Directions: Decide whether the following statements are True or False according to the text.

1. According to a recent analysis, expenditures on wound care, especially surgical wounds and diabetic ulcers, are far greater than we recognized.

2. With the advancements in science and technology, many aspects of wound care have been transformed to make it smarter, faster and more efficient.

3. The newly developed biofoam is bioabsorbable, flexible, durable and safe for

long-term use.

4. Inspired by his collaborators from Harvard and Purdue University, Sonkusale decided to develop a way to monitor wound healing in real time.

5. With the on-demand, smart solution of the bandage, doctors don't need to monitor the healing process of their patients.

6. Tamayol is excited about the bandage's potential, and he is optimistic about bringing it onto the market soon.

7. With lots of advancements put forward in the engineering world, we can easily get them into clinical practice.

8. Much of the research by Xudong Wang focuses on generating energy from the human body.

9. Having experimented on rats and pigs, Xudong Wang is now testing his bandage on humans.

10. It is likely that Xudong Wang's bandage can be proved effective to deal with burn wounds and help to minimize scar formation.

B. Directions: Answer the following questions according to your understanding of the text.

1. What is the focus of research by Jeffrey Catchmark and why does he focus his research on this?

2. How does the new material (the biofoam) take effect after it is placed within the traumatic wounds?

3. In which aspects can this new material (the biofoam) really impact our lives?

4. In what ways is Sonkusale's prototype bandage smart?

5. According to Sonkusale, what new technology makes it possible for him to design this smart, flexible and thin material that can serve as a bandage?

6. How can doctors provide treatments from afar with the smart bandage invented by Ali Tamayol?

7. What are the top concerns of patients and care providers respectively?

8. What are other therapeutic uses of Xudong Wang's new technology?

II. Vocabulary

Directions: Choose the best word or expression from the list given for each blank. Use each word or expression only once and make proper changes when necessary.

chronic	range	attribute	individualize	streamline
derive	acute	inspire	penetrate	harness

1. Another important _____ is the unique boiling point of helium (氦), which is lower than any other element.

2. Tetanus is the _____ bacterial disease caused by clostridium tetani.

3. We encourage them to remain active and mobile, and we _____ therapy according to specific needs.

4. There is no easy short-term solution to the country's _____ economic recession.

5. They are making efforts to _____ some of the administrative procedures, and improve human resource planning.

6. A child can become deeply absorbed in something, and _____ intense pleasure from that absorption.

7. The science of statistics tells us that positive correlations _____ from 0.0 to 1.0.

8. This method of cooking also permits heat to _____ evenly from both sides.

9. We must promote originality, _____ creativity and encourage innovation.

10. Let us _____ the magic of football in our quest for development and peace.

III. Topics for Discussion

1. Can you imagine some cases or scenarios where the smart bandage of Sonkusale can be applied? What other devices can be added or embedded in the bandage to make it more individualized in that case?

2. Two types of smart bandages are mentioned in the passage, one developed by Sonkusale, and the other by Tamayol. Can you list the similarities and differences between them?

3. What are the new technologies (or materials/devices) mentioned in the passage? Which one seems to be the most practicable to you?

Text B
Endoscopic Iliotibial Band Release during Hip Arthroscopy for Femoroacetabular Impingement Syndrome and External Snapping Hip had better Patient-Reported Outcomes: A Retrospective Comparative Study

Chunbao Li

Abstract

Purpose: To compare patient-reported outcomes (PROs) in patients with femoroacetabular impingement (FAI) syndrome and external snapping hip (ESH) treated with hip arthroscopy with or without endoscopic iliotibial band (ITB) release.

Methods: Cases with both FAI syndrome and ESH who had undergone surgical treatment were retrospectively analyzed. According to the primary surgical approaches chosen by patients themselves, the patients undergoing ITB release during hip arthroscopy for FAI syndrome were enrolled in the ITB-R group, while those undergoing hip arthroscopy without ITB release were assigned to the Non-ITB-R group. Patients with dysplasia, severe osteoarthritis, revision and bilateral surgery were excluded. Patient-reported outcomes (PROs) including international Hip Outcome Tool (iHOT-33), modified Harris Hip Score (mHHS), visual analog scale for pain (VAS-pain) and VAS-satisfaction, and the rates of achieving minimal clinically important difference (MCID), patient acceptable symptomatic state (PASS) and substantial clinical benefit (SCB) for the PROs at 2 years postoperatively were comparatively analyzed.

Results: The prevalence of ESH in FAI syndrome patients who had undergone hip arthroscopy in our institution was 4.9% (30 of 612 hips). The mean age at the time of surgery was 33.1 ± 6.9 years (ranging from 22 to 48 years). After exclusion, 16 patients (16 hips) were enrolled into ITB-R group and 11 patients (11 hips) into Non-ITB-R group. PROs including iHOT-33, mHHS, VAS-pain and VAS-satisfaction in patients in ITB-R group were better than those in Non-ITB-R group at two years postoperatively ($P=0.013$, 0.016, 0.002 and 0.005, respectively). The rates of achieving PASS for mHHS, PASS for VAS-pain and SCB for iHOT-33 of patients in ITB-R group were significantly better than those in Non-ITB-R group ($P=0.009$, 0.006 and 0.027, respectively).

Conclusions: Patients with both FAI syndrome and ESH undergoing ITB release during hip arthroscopy had better PROs than those undergoing hip arthroscopy without ITB release.

Femoroacetabular impingement (FAI) syndrome is the most common cause of hip pain in young and middle-aged adults. Prevalence of FAI syndrome among young, middle-aged Caucasian adults is approximately 3%, and higher in the athletic population. Hip arthroscopy has been increasingly used as a minimally invasive means of addressing FAI syndrome for the past two decades. It demonstrably gives FAI syndrome patients excellent pain relief and improvement in function.

Our clinical practice showed that several FAI syndrome patients also suffer from external snapping hip (ESH). Due to the complexity of the structures around the hip, FAI syndrome patients sometimes have extra-articular disorders, such as trochanteric bursitis, ESH or internal snapping hip, along with intra-articular injuries, such as labral tear and chondral injury. ESH is commonly caused by an enlarged or tight posterior portion of the iliotibial band (ITB) and a tight anterior border of the tendinous insertion of the gluteus maximus muscle. In addition, structure disorders of the hip such as dysplasia and coxa vara also frequently result in ESH. The mechanism of snapping comes as the ITB slides over and catches on the superior border of the greater trochanter of the femur with the flexion and extension of the hip during exercise or ordinary daily activities. Continuously presenting external snapping causes pain due to inflammatory thickening of the ITB and greater trochanteric bursitis.

A therapeutic schedule for FAI patients that also suffer from ESH lacks large-scale reporting and is inconsistent. Non-surgical measures of ESH, including anti-inflammatories, stretching, and avoidance of inciting activities, can provide patients with pain relief but have a poor effect on eliminating hip snapping. For refractory patients that do not respond to non-surgical treatments, surgical intervention such as open or endoscopic ITB release is an excellent alternative. Typically, FAI patients who also suffer from ESH can undergo endoscopic ITB release after intra-articular arthroscopic management is finished. Thus, it remains unclear whether patients with both FAI syndrome and ESH undergoing ITB release during hip arthroscopy might have a better outcome than the patients undergoing hip arthroscopy without ITB release.

The purpose of this study was to compare patient-reported outcomes (PROs) in patients with both FAI syndrome and ESH treated with hip arthroscopy with or without endoscopic iliotibial band (ITB) release. Our hypothesis was that patients with both FAI syndrome and ESH undergoing endoscopic ITB release for ESH during hip arthroscopy would have better PROs than those undergoing hip arthroscopy without ITB release.

The most important finding of our study was that patients with both FAI syndrome and ESH undergoing ITB release during hip arthroscopy had better PROs than those undergoing hip arthroscopy without ITB release, including iHOT-33, mHHS, VAS-pain and VAS-satisfaction (as well as more frequently to achieve PASS for mHHS, PASS for VAS-pain and SCB for iHOT-33). Our data also indicated that the prevalence of ESH in FAI patients in our specified cohort was 4.9% (30 in 612 hips) and that females might be more vulnerable to FAI and ESH concurrently.

The 4.9% incidence rate of EHS in the FAI cohort in our institution is very close to the one reported by Vap AR et al., which reviewed a cohort of 1,278 patients who underwent hip arthroscopy at their institution and found a prevalence of 7% of trochanteric bursitis in FAI patients. Due to the complex structure of the hip, extra-articular disorders such as hip snapping and trochanter bursitis are of interest to arthroscopic surgeons, as these conditions may affect the outcome of the hip arthroscopy in FAI patients. ESH is prevalent in active patients and often negatively affects their daily activities. FAI patients are more likely to get ESH due to their underlying hip condition, altered gait mechanics, pelvic muscular imbalance and lumbopelvic abnormality. Thus, the prevalence of ESH in FAI patients is higher than that in the normal population.

There is no consensus on therapeutic strategies for patients with both FAI and ESH. The primary intervention for ESH consists of rest and avoidance of activities that produce snapping. If snapping causes pain and affects daily activities, a local injection of steroids, oral anti-inflammatory medication and ITB stretching can be used to alleviate pain and improve activity. For refractory cases, surgical ITB release is the final solution. Many previous studies have shown that ITB release can relieve external hip pain and eliminate snapping, while being minimally invasive and having a low recurrence rate of snapping. Endoscopic ITB release has become the most favorable surgical treatment for ESH, as it not only relieves lateral hip pain at the greater trochanter, but also eliminates the snapping. Our study showed that patients with both FAI syndrome and ESH still developed snapping symptoms and had their daily activities affected. Thus, for FAI patients complicated with ESH who need hip arthroscopy, endoscopic

ITB release should be performed to prevent subsequent hip snapping.

In previous literature, some surgeons indicated that they performed ITB release after intra-articular operation was finished when the patients also had ESH or great trochanteric bursitis. Vap et al. also reported that for patients with FAI and great trochanteric bursitis, undergoing bursectomy with ITB release had no negative effect on hip arthroscopy outcomes and led to significant improvements in functional outcomes and patient satisfaction. However, studies mentioned above failed to mention whether endoscopic ITB release during hip arthroscopy would deliver a better outcome than hip arthroscopy without ITB release in patients with both FAI syndrome and ESH. Our study showed that the postoperative non-surgical treatment for ESH in patients in non-ITB-R group could not eliminate external snapping, and their PROs were worse than those of patients in ITB group. Snapping continued to disturb patients and led them to get subsequent ITB release surgery. Overall, their level of satisfaction was lower than tha of those who had ITB release performed during their primary hip surgery. Our study provides strong evidence that in FAI patients with ESH, ITB release should be performed during primary hip arthroscopy to maximize the outcome of hip arthroscopy and patient satisfaction.

The technique of surgical interventions for ESH has been developing for decades. Portion resection of ITB, Z-plasty technique or modified Z-plasty technique for lengthening ITB, cruciate or transverse incision on ITB for release were reported with good results. Currently, surgeons prefer endoscopic to open surgery for ITB release. Mitchell et al. reported an endoscopic ITB release technique using a cruciate incision on the ITB, 2cm horizontally and 2cm longitudinally, to release the tight ITB and expose the trochanteric bursa. However, we performed a larger transverse incision of the ITB to release the tight ITB. Typically, a 5-7cm incision thoroughly releases the ITB and perfectly exposes the trochanteric bursa. This transverse incision technique was performed in open surgery in the 1980s with a very good outcome. Zini et al. first reported in 2013 performing an endoscopic transverse incision to release ITB and showed that this technique for ITB release was safe and reproducible in ESH. There has been no evidence as to which technique is better.

We use transverse incision technique because it easily releases the ITB completely, unlike the cruciate incision technique where the cross-over point of vertical and horizontal incision has to be at an appropriate location. Additionally, a transverse incision diminishes the concern over residual inflammation caused by waggling of ITB tissue blades generated by the cruciate incision. We would like to emphasize that it is not necessary to establish another distal portal usually used in isolated endoscopic ITB release surgery, as the DALA portal is sufficient to perform the ITB release. Another detail of our technique is the management of the greater trochanter bursa. Although prior literature suggests that bursectomy was necessary to remove the inflammatory synovium of the bursa, we only did inflammatory synovium debridement on cases with severe bursitis and did nothing about cases with mild bursitis around the greater trochanter. It is very hard to say which technique is the best for addressing ESH. We believe that surgeons could choose one of these techniques to do ITB release for the patients with both FAI syndrome and external snapping base on surgeon's personal experience and inclination.

(This article is excepted from "Endoscopic Iliotibial Band Release during Hip Arthroscopy for Femoroacetabular Impingement Syndrome and External Snapping Hip had Better Patient-Reported Outcomes: A Retrospective Comparative Study" published in *The Journal of Arthroscopic and Related Surgery*, PMID: 33539977)

Words and Expressions

1. demonstrably: *adv.* in an obvious and provable manner 可论证地，明确地

2. inciting: *adj.* giving an incentive for action 刺激性的

3. alternative: *n.* a thing that you can choose to do or have out of two or more possibilities （两者或多者中）另种选择，替代方案

4. be inclined to: having a preference, disposition, or tendency 倾向于

5. concurrently: *adv.* existing or happening at the same time 同时地，并发地

6. consensus: *n.* general agreement among a group of people 一致的意见，共识

7. lateral: *adj.* relating to the sides of something, or moving in a sideways direction 侧面的，横向的

8. longitudinally: *adv.* in the direction of the length 纵向地

9. reproducible: *adj.* capable of being reproduced 可再生的，可繁殖的

10. transverse: *adj.* extending or lying across; in a crosswise direction 横向的，横断的

Medical Vocabulary

iliotibial band： 髂胫束

femoroacetabular impingement (FAI)： 股骨髋臼撞击综合征

dysplasia： 发育不良

osteoarthritis： 骨关节炎

bursitis： 滑囊炎

chondral： 软骨的

coxa vara： 髋关节内翻

bursectomy： 滑膜切除术

synovium： 滑膜

Exercise

Critical Thinking

The present study uses both retrospective and comparative study methods to reach its conclusion. Both methods are commonly used in medical studies. Have you ever used them (retrospective, comparative, or both) in your previous studies? If yes, can you brief those studies and share with us the advantages and disadvantages of such a method according to your own experiences?

Supplementary Reading

For more information on Wound Care and Pain Relief, please go to the following websites:

1. https://www.ncbi.nlm.nih.gov/pmc/articles/PMC3478916/

2. https://www.nursingtimes.net/clinical-archive/tissue-viability/strategies-to-reduce-or-eliminate-wound-pain-04-04-2014/

3. https://www.emedicinehealth.com/wound_care/article_em.htm

Unit Six　CBRN[1] Injuries

Text A
General Considerations in Management of Chemical Casualties

This article provides an overview of basic concepts that should be considered by medical personnel involved in the management of chemical weapons incidents. Planning and training of these personnel will be necessary for effective management of such incidents, particularly those involving a large number of chemical casualties whose arrival in surges at a medical support facility is likely to exceed its normal capacity.

Important challenges when dealing with a chemical weapons incident include:

1) Rapid agent detection and identification;

2) Hazard avoidance through adequate protection and decontamination, as well as cordons to control entry to and exit from the affected area;

3) Casualty decontamination, not only to reduce contact of the agent with the victim, but to avoid spreading contamination to medical treatment facilities; and

4) Triage and quick medical treatment, including specific antidote therapy at the site of the incident and at the hospital level to reduce morbidity and mortality. It is important to note that medical personnel may have to deal with mass casualties, some of whom may not even have been poisoned but who may have psychogenic symptoms.

Management of a chemical incident is an ongoing process that aims to reduce or avoid potential secondary losses, assure prompt and appropriate assistance to victims, and achieve rapid and effective recovery. A basic disaster management cycle addresses at least the following phases:

1) *Prevention and mitigation*: Actions are taken before the incident to prevent or minimise consequences through assessments of hazards and vulnerabilities.

2) *Preparedness*: Assessments from the first phase lead to the development of the plan to manage the chemical incident, including the acquisition of capabilities and training programmes. The plan should clearly integrate medical capabilities at the local, regional, and national levels. This may require the establishment of coordination agreements between different services and agencies so they can be integrated smoothly into the command and control system. Management plans should be as simple as possible and be clearly expressed, as complex plans may be difficult to implement.

3) *Response*: The emergency plan is put into practice in a real-time event. The response phase will depend on the preparedness phase.

4) *Recovery*: Finally, actions are taken to return to the pre-event situation. Such actions might include disposal of hazardous materials and remediation of the incident site, as well as further assistance to victims.

Medical management is important in all phases, although often these phases overlap and the duration of each one will vary depending on the nature and severity of the incident.

1. Detection (diagnosis)

When a CW incident takes place it is unlikely that, initially, first responders and medical personnel will know the identity of the agent, unless there is prior warning by intelligence or law enforcement sources. Moreover, results of unambiguous identification from laboratory identification of environmental and clinical samples will take time to reach medical personnel.

There are differing technologies available for rapid on-site detection and identification of CW agents. These include, among others:

Ion mobility spectrometry;

Flame photometry;

Colourimetric/enzyme methods;

Surface acoustic wave device;

Photoionisation;

Fourier transform infrared spectroscopy;

Raman spectroscopy; and

Gas chromatography/mass spectrometry.

All portable detection/identification devices, regardless of the technology used, sometimes yield false positives and false negatives due to their sensitivity and selectivity. Using detectors with one technology provides "provisional" detection, while using detectors of at least two different technologies provides a higher level of assurance, in particular if a colourimetric method or gas chromatography/mass spectrometry is one of the two techniques used or employed.

While most portable detection equipment detects nerve and blister agents, not all of them have capabilities to detect other CW agents. Also, most of these devices were developed for military scenarios, and while available in some emergency units, they may give false responses in civilian scenarios.

For all these reasons, including a lack of availability of detection equipment in some situations, as well as lack of sufficient sensitivity and specificity, information from the signs and symptoms of poisoned patients will most likely provide the first indication of use of chemical weapons.

Medical personnel should be familiar with the main clinical signs and symptoms necessary to determine a clinical diagnosis and start the triage process, assigning priority for decontamination and medical treatment. It is important to note that the nature and timing of these clinical manifestations will vary not only with the duration and concentration of exposure, but also with the route of exposure, which should be considered in the differential diagnosis and triage process. For example, nerve agents and cyanides (blood agents) absorbed by inhalation have rapid onset of effects and need immediate treatment.

Differential diagnosis should also consider the indirect effects of chemical exposure, including heat stress from wearing protective equipment, psychological effects, and even side effects from antidotes, especially in cases where exposure to an agent has not taken place but antidotes have been administered (for example, autoinjectors with nerve agent poisoning antidotes). Differential diagnosis and triage may also be complicated in cases of mixed casualties who have both conventional and chemical injuries.

2. Protection measures

Medical personnel are a critical resource in case of chemical attack causing a large number of casualties. As with other responders, it is important that they do not become victims themselves. Personal protective equipment (PPE)[2] is the first line of defence in a chemically contaminated environment. PPE comprises a respirator and protective clothing, including suitable gloves and boots. Respirators are especially important as generally CW agents have their greatest and most rapid effect via the respiratory system.

Commonly, medical personnel will deal with poisoned patients once they have been removed from the contaminated area and have been decontaminated. However, some first-responder services and agencies (for example, firefighters and law enforcement personnel) that enter the directly affected area may assign or attach medical personnel for their own support and to make an early medical assessment. In these cases PPE will prevent exposure to chemical agents through direct contact with victims' skin, mucosa, and clothing or by inhalation of a persisting vapour hazard (particularly in confined and enclosed spaces).

Medical management while using PPE will be made more difficult due to loss of vision, mobility, dexterity, and ability to communicate. Also, working with PPE increases metabolic work, which in turn increases heat production and prevents dissipation of the heat generated by the body, increasing the risk of heat stress. This may worsen in case of adverse environmental conditions like high temperatures, high humidity, and low wind velocity, which will increase sweating and rapid dehydration. Only individuals who are physically fit and have received appropriate training in PPE should intervene in incidents requiring its use.

The criteria used for the classification of PPE and PPE levels vary in different countries. One of the most frequently used, included in the OPCW[3]'s assistance and protection training courses, is the US Environmental Protection Agency (EPA)[4] four-level classification (Table 6-1). These levels differ in respiratory and skin protection, and selection is based on the type of agent, toxicity, and concentration.

Table 6-1　Classification of PPE Used by the US EPA

Level of Protection	Respiratory Protection	Skin Protection	Scenario
A	Pressure demand full-facepiece self-contained breathing apparatus (SCBA)[5]	Fully-encapsulated chemical-resistant suit; Chemical-resistant inner and external gloves and boots/shoes	Unknown agent; Known agent and significant hazard of exposure (for example, high concentrations, risk of splash, immersion).
B	Pressure demand full-facepiece SCBA	Non-encapsulated hooded chemical-resistant clothing; Chemical-resistant inner and outer gloves and boots/shoes.	Agent known and significant, respiratory protection required (but less skin protection); Atmosphere contains less that 19.5% oxygen.
C	Full-face or half-mask air-purifying respirator (APR)[6]	Non-encapsulated hooded chemical-resistant clothing; Chemical resistant inner and outer gloves and boots/shoes.	Agent and environment concentration known to be removed by an APR; Skin contact with known agent is non-hazardous and significant transdermal absorption does not occur; Atmosphere contains at least 19.5% oxygen.
D	None	Common work uniform	No known hazard

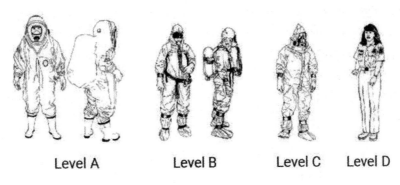

Level A　　　Level B　　　Level C　　Level D

Figure 6-1　PPE levels used by the US EPA

Level A in the EPA classification should be used if the identity of the agent is unknown, or if there is risk of inhalation of a high concentration of toxic agents or risk of significant skin or mucosae damage. It consists of a fully encapsulated, vapour-tight, chemical-resistant suit, chemical-resistant inner and outer gloves, chemical-resistant shoes or boots, and a self-contained breathing apparatus (SCBA). In case of leaks, positive pressure will allow air flow from the inside to the outside, but not from the outside to the inside.

Level B protection is used when the highest level of respiratory protection is needed (including atmospheres deficient in oxygen), but a lesser degree of skin protection is required. Thus, it includes the SCBA, but non-encapsulated suits can be used.

Level C has the same skin protection as Level B, but uses an air-purifying respirator (APR) instead of an SCBA. There are different classes and types of commercially available filters with established colour-coding systems to indicate the chemical substances against which they can be used.

Level D is the common work uniform. Surgical masks, gowns, and gloves commonly used by medical personnel are also considered as Level D. These should not be worn on any site where respiratory or skin CW agent hazards exist.

3. Hospital management

Hospitals need to be integrated in the disaster management plan. This will provide adequacy of patient evacuation based not only on their proximity to the affected area, but also on their capability to receive patients, which should be continually updated during the response phase in order to maintain a balanced patient distribution. Good communication will also ensure adequate ambulance transport to suitable reception areas. Integration of all medical treatment facilities in the management system will also ensure dissemination of the identification of the CW agent, once it is conclusively verified by laboratory tests. Thus, adequate medical treatment, including antidotal therapy, can be provided.

Hospitals should also have their own emergency plans. Once activated, security personnel should control the access of people and vehicles to the hospital and direct them to the reception area. It is possible that contaminated patients may arrive by their own means, and a decontamination corridor (similar to that of the warm zone will have to be deployed, commonly outside the emergency department or in a previously established area. Hospital staff entering into contact with potentially contaminated patients should use PPE. Level C protection is commonly sufficient.

(This article is excerpted from *Practical Guide for Medical Management of Chemical Warfare Casualties*)

Notes

1. CBRN: chemical, biological, radiological and nuclear 化学、生物、放射和核

2. personal protective equipment (PPE): protective equipment, including protective clothing and protective mask, especially designed to protect personnel against hazards caused by extreme changes in physical environment, dangerous working conditions, or enemy actions 个人防护装备

3. OPCW: The Organisation for the Prohibition of Chemical Weapons (OPCW) is the implementing body for the Chemical Weapons Convention, which entered into force on 29 April 1997. The OPCW, with its 193 Member States, oversees the global endeavor to permanently and verifiably eliminate chemical weapons. 禁止化学武器组织

4. US Environmental Protection Agency (EPA): an agency of the United States federal government whose mission is to protect human and environmental health. Headquartered in Washington, D.C., the EPA is responsible for creating standards and laws promoting the health of individuals and the environment. The EPA regulates the manufacturing, processing, distribution, and use of chemicals and other pollutants. 美国环境保护署

5. self-contained breathing apparatus (SCBA): a breathable compressed air supplying respiratory device. The term self-contained means that the SCBA is not dependent on a remote supply of breathing gas. Instead, the breathing air source is designed to be carried by the user. It is typically used by the firefighters and rescue workers while operating in areas of immediate danger to life and health. 自给式呼吸器

6. air-purifying respirator (APR): works by removing gases, vapors, aerosols (droplets and solid particles), or a combination of contaminants from the air through the use of filters, cartridges, or canisters. These respirators do not supply oxygen and therefore cannot be used in an atmosphere that is oxygen-deficient or immediately dangerous to life or health. 空气净化呼吸器

Words and Expressions

1. yield: *v.* to produce or provide something, for example, a profit, result or crop 出产（作物）；产生（收益、效益等）

2. mitigation: *n.* a reduction in the unpleasantness, seriousness, or painfulness of something 减轻，缓和

3. remediation: *n.* the action of remedying something, of correcting an error or fault 补救，矫正

4. overlap: *v.* if two events overlap or overlap each other, they involve some of the same subjects, people, or periods of time. （时间、内容上）部分重叠

5. unambiguous: *adj.* clear in meaning; that can only be understood in one way 意思清楚的，明确的，无歧义的

6. dissemination: *n.* the opening of a subject to widespread discussion and debate 发散，散播

7. provisional: *adj.* not final or fully worked out or agreed upon 临时性的，假定的

8. scenario: *n.* a setting, in particular for a work of art or literature 情景，场

9. specificity: *n.* the quality of being specific rather than general 特异性

10. inhalation: *n.* the act of inhaling; the drawing in of air (or other gases) as in breathing 吸入

11. administer: *v.* to give drugs, medicine, etc. to somebody 给予，施用（药物等）

12. dexterity: *n.* skill in using your hands or your mind （手）灵巧，熟练；（思维）敏捷，灵活

13. dissipation: *n.* the process of disappearing or of making something disappear 消散；驱散

14. velocity: *n.* the speed of something in a particular direction （沿某一方向的）速度

15. intervene: *v.* (in something) to become involved in a situation in order to improve or help it 出面；介入

16. encapsulate: *v.* to enclose in a capsule or other small container 压缩

17. leak: *n.* liquid or gas that escapes through a hole in something 泄漏出的液体（或

气体）

18. deficient: *adj.* not having enough of something, especially something that is essential 缺乏的；不足的

19. proximity: *n.* the state of being near somebody/something in distance or time （时间或空间）接近，邻近，靠近

Medical Vocabulary

specific antidote: 特效解毒剂

psychogenic: 精神性的

ion mobility spectrometry: 离子迁移光谱法

flame photometry: 火焰光度法

clourimetric / enzyme method: 比色法/酶法

surface acoustic wave device: 表面声波器件

photoionisation: 光化电离

Fourier transform infrared spectroscopy: 傅里叶变换红外光谱法

Raman spectroscopy: 拉曼光谱法

gas chromatography / mass spectrometry: 气相色谱法/质谱分析法

blister agent: 糜烂性毒剂

differential diagnosis: 临床鉴别诊断

nerve agent: 神经性毒剂

cyanide: 氰化物

heat stress: 热应激

Exercises

I. Reading Comprehension

A. Directions: Decide whether the following statements are True or False according to the text.

1. In a CW incident, all the casualties the medial personnel deal with must have been poisoned.

2. Disaster management plans should be as complex as possible so that everything can be taken into consideration.

3. It is highly possible that first responders will know the identity of the CW agent at the very beginning of their action without prior warning from other sources.

4. To ensure a "confirmed" detection of CW agents, both the colourimetric method and the gas chromatography / mass spectrometry have to be employed.

5. Some of the portable detection equipment can detect CW agents besides nerve and blister agents.

6. Nerve agents should be given priority for medical treatment because they are absorbed

by inhalation and have rapid onset of effects.

7. Chemical-resistant suits are especially important as generally CW agents have the most rapid effect via direct contact with the victim.

8. Medical personnel are not supposed to enter the directly affected area in any case.

9. For Level C protection, we can use APR with different filters bought from the market to deal with different chemical substances.

10. In case of emergency, all vehicles, including ambulances, have to transport to the reception area of the hospital.

B. Directions: Answer the following questions according to your understanding of the text.

1. What are the important challenges when dealing with a CW incident?

2. What are the 4 phases included in the basic disaster management cycle?

3. Can you list at least 5 different technologies available for rapid on-site detection and identification of CW agents?

4. How to avoid false positives and false negatives during the detection of CW agents?

5. Why is it important for medical personnel to be familiar with the main clinical signs and symptoms necessary to determine a clinical diagnosis and start the triage process?

6. What is the first line of defence in a chemically contaminated environment? What does it usually consist of?

7. What are the disadvantages of using PPE?

8. Which level of protection (in the EPA classification) is used when the highest level of respiratory and skin protection is needed? And what devices are usually included?

II. Vocabulary

Directions: Choose the best word or expression from the list given for each blank. Use each word or expression only once and make proper changes when necessary.

surge	unambiguous	overlap	administer
deficient	vulnerability	intervene	yield

1. The _____ in car sales was regarded as an encouraging pointer to an improvement in the economy.

2. This research has been in progress since 1961 and has _____ a great number of positive results.

3. The minister said she would give a clear and _____ statement on the future of the coal industry at the earliest possible opportunity.

4. If there were a breakdown of law and order, the army might be tempted to _____.

5. Our jobs _____ slightly, which sometimes causes difficulties.

6. Taking long-term courses of certain medicines may increase _____ to infection.

7. They believe such a diet which includes no products from animal sources can

be _____ in many of the necessary vitamins and minerals our bodies need.

8. The physician may prescribe but not _____ the drug.

III. Topics for Discussion

1. Can you illustrate how the disaster management cycle works with a more detailed example (i.e. how it works in an earthquake or an epidemic)?

2. Discuss with your partner about the responsibilities of medical personnel during a CW incident.

3. What are the greatest challenges for health care providers in a CW incident?

Text B
Medical Management of Radiation Injuries: Current Approaches

M. E. Berger

Introduction

New technologies and research during the past 20 years have provided a greater understanding of the complex nature of radiation injury at molecular, cellular, tissue and organ system levels. The experience gained both in radiation therapy and in medical care of radiation accident patients has enabled development and use of new assessment and treatment modalities and provided more information about complications and numerous problems yet to be solved. Little can be done currently to prevent reproductive and apoptotic death of cells after radiation injury, but current therapy has potential to facilitate production of certain cells, provide replacement therapy for lost haematopoietic cells, minimize infectious complications, minimize fibrosis formation and improve supportive care.

Although radiation accidents are not common, human error, failure to follow safety precautions and inadequate control/regulation of radiation sources have led to deaths and significant exposures among workers and members of the public.

Physicians practising occupational medicine may be involved in immediate assessment and care of radiation accident victims. Under ordinary circumstances, they would not be involved in the treatment phase of the acute radiation syndrome (ARS) or serious local injuries, although they might be called on to explain procedures or prognoses to patients and their families. Their knowledge of triage, assessment, initial diagnostic methods and general treatment protocols, however, would be of great value in any radiation accident or incident involving harm to individuals. This paper will review some current approaches to triage, assessment, therapy and supportive care of irradiated victims. The psychological aspects of radiation accidents, although very important, are beyond the scope of this paper.

Initial assessment and diagnosis

Four factors are critical determinants in the initial medical management of victims presenting at a hospital or clinic following an accidental or malevolent act involving radiological or nuclear materials:

1. The number of victims involved. The ability to assess, diagnose and provide initial therapy may be compromised when large numbers of patients arrive for treatment. Triage is essential when personnel and material resources are scarce.

2. The presence/absence of thermal or conventional injuries. In incidents involving thermal or conventional injuries, along with total body or large volume partial body irradiation (i.e., combined injury), initial triage, assessment and treatment must first focus on the conventional injuries present. Diagnosis of the ARS and estimates of severity are made after the immediate lifesaving treatment of trauma, since the radiation injury does not present immediate life-threatening complications.

3. The amount of time that has elapsed since the exposure(s) occurred is important since victims presenting soon after being irradiated (i.e., minutes to 48h) will have signs and symptoms and laboratory results that are different from those found in patients presenting days or weeks after exposures. Late presenting patients are likely to be sicker, with problems such as infectious complications, mucositis and/or painful skin lesions.

4. The presence of radioactive contaminants on the victim(s). A good rule of thumb is that most of the external contamination is removed by simply removing the victim's clothing. Decontamination (washing) of the skin of uninjured persons with external contamination should be completed at the earliest possible time, and prior to hospital admission. Injured persons can be decontaminated at the hospital or clinic once they are medically stable. Identification of the radionuclide(s) involved is important since proper treatment of internal contamination depends on knowing the specific element(s) involved.

Therapy in the prodromal phase

Patients with combined injuries should have serious trauma or burns evaluated and treated promptly according to conventional protocols. Necessary surgery should be completed within 24-36h of exposure. All blood or blood products used should be leuko-reduced and irradiated to 25 Gy as a means of minimizing the risk of developing graft-versus-host-disease. Once patients are stable, they should be assessed and treated for the ARS. These patients will become pancytopenic and immunocompromised, and healing of wounds will be delayed. Prognosis is generally poor for patients with combined injuries. Survival depends upon the type and severity of trauma, as well as upon the radiation dose.

Assessment and therapy in the latent and manifest illness phases

Except in special circumstances, treatment for radiation injury is not likely to be needed for patients having doses <1 Gy. Victims of a mass-casualty incident having estimated doses >10 Gy, and those with serious combined injuries, should have supportive care. If resources are available or if transfer to an unaffected hospital can be arranged, additional treatment can be provided. It is worth noting that many individuals seeking medical attention following a nuclear or radiological incident would not actually have been exposed to a significant radiation dose. Psychological support should be available for these individuals.

Prevention and treatment of infections

Recovery from the haematopoietic syndrome is dependent upon the ability to prevent or successfully treat infection in the immune-compromised patient. Depending on dose, the nadir of the leukocyte count is not reached for a matter of days to weeks after a victim is irradiated. This delay allows time to clear up existing infections, close skin wounds and treat mucositis prior to the onset of neutropenia. Most organisms are acquired from food, water and air, so precautions with food and water, restriction of contacts, use of laminar airflow or other controlled ventilation rooms, a protective environment and restriction of invasive procedures are desirable.

The severity of an infection in the ARS patient is dependent on the virulence of the infectious agent, the number of infectious organisms, the humoral and cell-mediated responses of the body and the presence of sufficient and effective phagocytic action within the body. The absolute neutrophil count is the most important and readily available measure of susceptibility to infection. Extreme neutropenia with absolute neutrophil counts of 500 cells/mme3 (0.500 × 10e9 cells/l) predicts impending infection. Febrile neutropenic patients require immediate intensive antibiotic treatment.

Infections are a significant problem in the gastrointestinal syndrome. Loss of the mucosal barrier allows translocation of commensal bacteria to the liver and spleen, with the possibility of a fatal septicaemia. Quinolone antibiotics have been effective in controlling these systemic infections because of their ability to eradicate species of Enterobacteriaceae. Quinolone-resistant organisms of the species Streptococcus may cause secondary infections.

Stimulation of new cell production

Treatment with a haematopoietic growth factor (GM-CSF, G-CSF or peg G-CSF) is recommended with radiation doses between 3 and 10 Gy, or as soon as the definite fall in the ALC below baseline (~2,000 lymphocytes) and a continued fall in follow-up of ALCs is noted. Growth factor treatment should be initiated in the first 24h for optimal efficacy.

Haematopoietic growth factors have also been developed to stimulate the production of megakaryocytes. Interleukin-11 is the only one of these currently being used. Erythropoietin has not been used in radiation accidents. Thrombocytopenia and anaemia can be significant in ARS patients and can be life threatening if radiation doses are high, if there are combined injuries or if the cutaneous syndrome is present.

Management of gastrointestinal injuries

Antibiotic administration does not prevent severe radiation-induced mucositis. Research has shown that GM-CSF (topically or subcutaneously) does not relieve the symptoms. Sucralfate mouthwash has been shown to be of benefit in decreasing the sensitivity and discomfort. Repifermin and palifermin [both recombinant human keratinocyte growth factor (KGF)] have shown promise in reducing the duration and severity of mucositis in radiotherapy patients when given prior to or after therapy. Their use in accidents has not been documented. Sharp has pointed out that the use of haematopoietic growth factors has incidental beneficial effects on mucositis and the gastrointestinal (GI) syndrome, because the increase in neutrophils is associated with a decrease in infections.

The effects of a significant irradiation (>9 Gy) of the abdominal area vary with time. Minutes to hours after exposure, symptoms include nausea, vomiting, diarrhoea and possibly abdominal cramps. Hours to 2 days post-exposure, there is diarrhoea and delayed gastric emptying. Days to weeks later there is persistent diarrhoea, malabsorption, severe fluid and electrolyte imbalances and septicaemia. The prognosis associated with the GI syndrome is poor.

Haematopoietic cell replacement therapy

The loss of rapidly dividing, undifferentiated cells of the bone marrow results in deficiencies in all the formed elements of the blood. Haematopoietic stem cells are available for replacement from bone marrow donor, peripheral blood (PB) or umbilical cord blood. Stem cell transplants are commonly used in haematology and oncology.

Consideration for bone marrow transplant (BMT) should be for persons whose exposure was relatively uniform and in the dose range of 7-10 Gy. In most cases, persons with serious trauma or thermal injury should not be candidates for BMT. Bone marrow from a human leukocyte antigen (HLA) identical sibling or family member is preferable for a stem cell transplant, but often is not available. A search for a non-related matching donor is time consuming. Fliedner has defined the target dose of CD34+ bone marrow cells for engraftment of an HLA-matched allogenic BMT in the recipient as $3 \times 10e6$ CD34+ cells/kg body weight. Attempts to stimulate production of cells with G-CSF shortly after a BMT appear to increase the risk of GVHD.

PB stem cells can be mobilized in an HLA-matched donor by pre-treatment with growth factor (G-CSF) prior to harvesting. The mobilization process requires ~4 days, but once PB is infused, engraftment and haematopoietic recovery occurs faster than with a BMT. PB grafts provide 10 times more T and B cells than marrow grafts, and as a result, PB recipients have fewer infections than those receiving BMT. AMD 3100, a chemokine receptor antagonist that is still in Phase 1 trials, appears to induce rapid mobilization of CD34+ within hours of its administration, with minimal side effects.

Umbilical cord blood is readily available, and acquiring it presents no risk to the donor. The recipient's risk of developing GVHD from a cord blood stem cell transplant is low, even with some HLA mismatch. A cord blood transplant contains a relatively small number of cells available for transplant, and this is a distinct disadvantage. In addition, engraftment takes longer. Davey has documented an average of 28 days for engraftment in children given cord blood, with a range of 11-60.

Management of skin injury

Treatment focuses on prevention of injury and infection in the involved area, prevention of further vasculature insult, pain control, fostering an acute wound-healing environment and minimizing fibrosis. Recommendations typically include cessation of smoking, nutritional supplements of vitamins A, C and E, use of pentoxifylline to decrease the viscosity of blood and to improve its flow, treatment of infection and, when necessary, careful surgical debridement of devitalized tissue. Various topical drugs such as silver sulfadiazine and steroids are often used for moist reactions. Integra®, a bilaminate skin substitute, has been used with success to cover wounds and facilitate formation of granulation tissue in preparation for skin grafting. Recombinant human platelet-derived growth factor (becaplermin) and KGF, not yet approved for radiation injuries, may be used to foster granulation and epithelialization. Hom and Manivel reported the successful use of becaplermin in treating a 12-year-old, previously irradiated problem wound. Milanov advises surgical treatment with aggressive debridement and immediate coverage with well-vascularized skin flaps to provide rapid healing and return of function. Reduction of fibrosis formation in chronic radiation wounds has been achieved with the use of injected interferon gamma.

The cutaneous syndrome that involves an extensive area of skin and possibly deep tissue injury results in systemic problems such as those found with large area thermal burns. The dangers of infection, haemorrhage, anaemia, endogenous intoxication, disseminated intra-vascular coagulation and multi-organ failure are always present. If a patient has both the cutaneous syndrome and the haematopoietic syndrome, the prognosis is very poor. Barabonova reported that severe cutaneous syndrome dramatically affected the survival of patients with the ARS following the Chernobyl accident. It was the main cause of death in more than half the lethal cases. Collaboration of haematologists, burn specialists, radiation oncologists, radiation medicine specialists, infectious disease specialists, psychologists and specialists in pain control is needed for the complex treatment of these patients.

Treatment of internal contamination

Internal contamination with radionuclides can occur by inhalation, ingestion, absorption through a wound or intact skin and injection. It is important to treat internal contamination promptly, preferably within the first several hours after exposure. Treatment of life-threatening trauma, however, takes priority. Internal contamination does not usually occur without external contamination being present, except in unusual circumstances (i.e. ingestion of water or foodstuffs contaminated by a malevolent act, or inhalation and/or ingestion of contaminants following a serious reactor or nuclear weapon incident). Radionuclides react chemically exactly the same as their stable counterparts and therefore the body does not distinguish between one or the other, metabolizing them both exactly the same. Treatment varies with each specific element involved, so it becomes extremely important to identify each contaminant. Identification by bio-assay is slow and a specimen can be easily contaminated.

Identification by whole-body counting is limited by residual skin contamination, variable chest wall thicknesses and other technical factors.

Careful questioning may result in identification of the contaminant in an occupational setting. In addition, a careful investigation by the health physicist or radiation safety officer will make the identification and/or verify the history provided by the patient. A body survey, to rule out external contamination should be done. Swabs of the right and left nares, nasal blows and sputum samples should be collected in separate containers.

When wounds are found to be contaminated, they should be thoroughly irrigated and cleansed to prevent further radiation exposure and internal absorption. The contamination should preferably be reduced to background levels, but this is seldom possible. Treatment to reduce the retention in the tissues is required.

An estimate of the amount of internal uptake must be made after identification of the specific radionuclide. Small amounts may not require treatment. The annual limit of intake (ALI) is a value that can be determined by the health physicist or radiation safety officer. If the value exceeds the ALI and the patient is a young person, then treatment may be considered. In older persons (>60 years), higher limits may be tolerated.

Summary

Early diagnosis and dose assessment are important when persons are accidentally or intentionally injured by ionizing radiation. Administration of haematopoietic growth factors can minimize the period of neutropenia in the ARS patient. Prevention and control of infection and excellent supportive care are essential to survival. The presence of gastrointestinal and/or cutaneous syndromes increases the chance of significant morbidity and mortality. Replacement of stem cells using bone marrow, PB or cord blood stem cells may benefit selected cases. Immune reconstitution and persistent thrombocytopenia continue to be problematic in treatment, as does the cutaneous syndrome. Nevertheless, current approaches to treatment facilitate survival at doses once thought to be lethal.

(This article is excepted from "Medical management of radiation injuries: current approaches" published in *Occupational Medicine*, PMID: 16641501)

Words and Expressions

1. compromise: *v.* to expose or make liable to danger, suspicion, or disrepute 使受到怀疑，使陷入危险，损害，破坏

2. elapse: *v.* (of time) to pass or go by 消逝，时间过去

3. a matter of: no more than (a specified period of time) 大约，左右

4. virulence: *n.* the severity or harmfulness of a disease or poison 毒性，毒力

5. susceptibility: *n.* the state or fact of being likely or liable to be influenced or harmed by a particular thing 敏感性，易感性

6. impending: *adj.* (of an event regarded as threatening or significant) about to happen;

forthcoming 即将发生的

7. undifferentiated: *adj.* not different or differentiated 无差别的，一致的

8. deficiency: *n.* a lack or shortage 缺乏，不足

9. sibling: *n.* each of two or more children or offspring having one or both parents in common; a brother or sister 兄弟姐妹

10. devitalize: *v.* to deprive of strength and vigor 使失去生命（devitalized: *adj.* 灭活的）

11. malevolent: *adj.* having or showing a wish to do evil to others 恶毒的，恶意的

12. counterpart: *n.* a person or thing holding a position or performing a function that corresponds to that of another person or thing in another place 对应的人或物

13. residual: *adj.* remaining after the greater part or quantity has gone 剩余的，残留的

Medical Vocabulary

acute radiation syndrome (ARS): 急性放射综合征

mucositis: 黏膜炎

radionuclide: 放射性核素

pancytopenic: 各类血细胞减少；全血细胞减少症

phagocytic: 噬菌作用的，噬菌细胞的

neutrophil: 中性粒细胞

neutropenia: 中性粒细胞减少症

septicaemia: 败血症

quinolone: 喹诺酮类

enterobacteriaceae: 肠杆菌科

streptococcus: 链球菌属

megakaryocytes: 巨核细胞

interleukin: 白细胞介素

erythropoietin: 促红细胞生成素

thrombocytopenia: 血小板减少症

cutaneous: 皮肤的

Exercise

Critical Thinking

Of all the approaches to triage, assessment, therapy and supportive care of irradiated victims mentioned in the passage, which have you had personal experiences with? Can you share with us your observations in that experience as to the problems with the present approach or practice? Even if you don't have any personal experiences, talk about the problems to be solved in the medical treatment of radiation injuries and the possible solutions to them in the future with the development of science and technology.

Supplementary Reading

For more information on CBRN Injuries, please go to the following websites:

1. https://ckapfwstor001.blob.core.usgovcloudapi.net/pfw-images/dbimages/Chem%20F M.pdf

2. https://biotech.law.lsu.edu/blaw/bluebook/Mmbch4AdobePDFVer4-02.pdf

3. https://ckapfwstor001.blob.core.usgovcloudapi.net/pfw-images/borden/nuclearwarfare /chap3chapter3.pdf

Unit Seven　Biosafety and Emergency Response

Text A
Medical Readiness: the Future of Medical Logistics

Brig. Gen. Michael B. Lalor

When the newly-organized Army Medical Logistics Command (AMLC) was activated last September, my focus was clear: prepare the organization to provide medical materiel and data from the strategic support area (SSA) to deliver effects at the tactical point of need in support of the operational force. Knowing we would soon operate in a contested multi-domain environment, we needed to rapidly improve our ability and capacity to deliver those effects.

Organizational change is never easy, especially the kind we were undertaking to systemically reform operational medical logistics. We expected long days, bumpy roads, and obstacles along the way. What none of us ever truly anticipated was a global pandemic. Less than six months into the command's development, we found ourselves at the center of the Army's support to the whole-of-government response to the novel coronavirus. AMLC continued throughout the summer to provide medical materiel to support ongoing and future operations across multiple global combatant commands.

COVID-19 is not the battle we forecasted but it provides us with a unique opportunity to test our ability to deliver effects from the SSA in a contested, real-world environment.

Developing the Army's Home for Medical Logistics since October 2018, we have witnessed a period of significant change as Army Medicine realigned delivery of fixed-site healthcare under the Defense Health Agency (DHA). This included the restructuring of US Army Medical Research and Materiel Command (USAMRMC) and the creation of AMLC.

Over a nine-month span, the Army reorganized and inactivated USAMRMC. Headquarters, Department of the Army, Execution Order 013-19 called for the immediate transfer of USAMRMC to US Army Materiel Command (AMC)[1]. A subsequent operations order 19-121 directed that USAMRMC "reorganizes to ensure compliance with Army future force modernization" and "develops a detailed plan to transfer medical research and development/program management to Army Futures Command." By June 1, 2019, MRMC was redesignated to US Army Medical Research and Development Command (MRDC) under Army Futures Command (AFC)[2].

To support operational medical logistics and forces in the field, the order also called for the creation of AMLC, a direct-report unit to AMC, which was activated on Sept. 17, 2019. The new AMLC was formed as a headquarters over three medical logistics subcommands: US Army Medical Materiel Agency, US Army Medical Materiel Center-Korea (USAMMC-K), and US Army Medical Materiel Center-Europe (USAMMC-E).

The creation of AMLC was part of several larger Army Medicine reform efforts to ensure medical readiness, support wartime requirements, and enhance the quality of care for soldiers and their families. Additionally, the Army sought to centralize medical logistics with the other sustainment functions inherent within AMC.

AMLC generates medical materiel readiness for the Army. Partnered with multiple stakeholders, AMLC ensures medical forces have the specialized equipment and materiel needed to continue the best care for soldiers, on and off the battlefield. AMLC sustains health services support for the operational Army units and joint forces, in support of large-scale combat operations (LSCO), through integrated medical materiel distribution, forward-positioned stocks, centralized medical materiel management, and data management.

Sustaining Strategic Support Area Operations

Today, AMLC serves as the Army's primary medical logistics and sustainment command. It provides strategic oversight of medical materiel within the Army prepositioned stocks (APS), forward-positioned stocks, operational projects, and medical maintenance operations located across four continents. AMLC supports AMC across four lines of effort within the SSA construct:

Industrial Base Readiness:

1. Provide sustainment-level repair, calibration, and recapitalization of medical equipment and medical special purpose test, measurement, and diagnostic equipment (TMDE-SP).

2. Deploy medical maintenance experts to operational environments to provide forward repair and maintenance support.

Strategic Power Projection:

1. Manage and sustain medical APS, forward-positioned stocks, and other medical materiel readiness programs.

2. Provide forward-operating optical fabrication, including standard issue and frame-of-choice glasses, inserts for gas masks and eye protection, and flight goggles for pilots.

3. Coordinate medical foreign military sales (FMS) in collaboration with US Department of State to strengthen our allied partners and ensure interoperability.

Supply Availability and Equipment Readiness:

1. Oversee the distribution of medical materiel (e.g., supplies, equipment, and assemblages) across the Army and joint medical forces.

2. Distribute vaccines and provide cold chain management training.

3. Support medical materiel quality control and hazard recall messaging.

4. Provide theater-level medical logistics support to Army and joint medical forces.

Data Analytics and Logistics Information Readiness:

1. Facilitate the Army's transition from the legacy medical logistics enterprise resource planning system (ERP) into Global Combat Support System-Army (GCSS-Army), to be completed no later than the end of fiscal year (FY) 2022.

2. Manage and update the medical materiel catalog.

3. Provide technical business support and record system training.

Fighting COVID-19

The first confirmed US case of the highly-contagious novel coronavirus was Jan. 21. By March 11, the World Health Organization (WHO) declared a global pandemic. For many Americans, this was the start of the battle. At AMLC, the fight began weeks earlier.

Theater Support Outside the Continental US

Medical Materiel Distribution. As cases began to increase within the US, AMLC was called to provide defense support of civil authorities (DSCA) through US Army North (USARNORTH)[3] as the joint forces land component command for US Northern Command (USNORTHCOM).

By March, AMLC teams distributed medical supplies for three Army hospital centers supporting New York and Washington states, two of the states initially hit hardest by COVID-19. This mission included support to Army medical professionals from 531st Hospital Center, from Fort Campbell, Kentucky, 627th Hospital, from Fort Carson, Colorado, and 9th Hospital Center, from Fort Hood, Texas. AMLC's unit deployment packages (UDPs) included potency and dated items tailored to each medical team's needs. These included everything from syringes and suction tubes to blood products and oxygen, intended to bolster these units' capabilities to deliver health care support where it was needed most.

Leveraging Army Prepositioned Stocks. Meanwhile, AMLC continued to provide worldwide support to the pandemic response. In Europe, AMLC issued medical materiel out of Army prepositioned stocks—including ventilators, patient monitors and hospital beds—for use at Landstuhl Regional Medical Center, Germany. We also issued field hospital sets to several locations overseas, including the USCENTCOM[4] area of operations, to augment Army capacity across the globe. AMLC prepositioned ventilators and ventilator resupply kits at various locations stateside for USNORTHCOM.

Integration Across the Army Sustainment Enterprise. Medical logistics is a lean specialty. In order to accomplish the mission, especially during COVID-19, Army Medicine had to integrate and synchronize efforts with others. This is where the creation of AMLC and its nesting as a major subordinate command under AMC really paid off. Inside AMC, integration and synchronization with the other direct reporting units and teammates helped AMLC mitigate shortfalls and gaps with storage, manpower, and distribution capability while providing unique capabilities in support of the medical maintenance mission.

Collaboration with Joint Partners and Key Stakeholders. The Army rarely deploys alone, so coordination among all military services and interoperability with allied partners is essential. AMLC routinely coordinates directly with:

1. Defense Logistics Agency-Troop Support (DLA-TS) for management of strategic medical materiel acquisition, distribution, and readiness programs.

2. Army Futures Command (AFC) and US Army Medical Research and Development Command (USAMRDC) to integrate logistics life-cycle management functions with program management functions and activities for development and delivery of sustainable materiel solutions

3. Defense Health Agency (DHA) in its execution of defense medical logistics programs and shared services, such as materiel standardization and data management

4. Defense Medical Logistics Enterprise and US Army Medical Command/Office of the Surgeon General for collaborative forums and initiatives to promote materiel standardization and joint interoperability

5. Army Service Component Commands and Combatant Commands for development and execution of MEDLOG portion of health service support plans

6. US Forces Command (FORSCOM) and its subordinate commands for medical force modernization and readiness, and installation-level medical supply, maintenance, and optical fabrication

During the fight against COVID-19, these established relationships became invaluable. Multiple resources, from hand sanitizer to test kits to PPE, quickly became in short supply. AMLC participated in joint priority allocation boards and collaborated with stakeholders to orchestrate the deliberate, needs-based delivery of medical materiel.

Rebuilding Capacity. Sustaining any long fight takes forward-thinking strategy and sustaining the fight against COVID-19 is no different. To date, AMLC has established enhanced processes to rapidly replenish potency and dated items, as well as expendables such as tubing on ventilators. A key part of this sustainment effort includes contracts with vendors and DLA-TS that gives us procurement speed and flexibility.

We've also had to think creatively about how we field and sustain items. Traditionally, we are a travel team. Our model called for us to physically go to a unit or deployment location, projecting our MLSTs to inventory and issue items. In a contested environment, COVID-19 travel restrictions forced us to change our playbook.

We hosted virtual training seminars online and produced maintenance tip sheets for many medical devices to boil down the most critical details for troubleshooting these items. We're sharing these products directly with medical maintainers and units around the globe. Our website also serves as a repository for the tip sheets and dozens of frequently asked questions to support the medical maintenance community.

We implemented "telemaintenance" virtually connecting maintainers with units in the field to assist with troubleshooting and repairing complicated medical devices. While it's only in its early stages, we believe this effort will have an incredible impact on our ability to extend our resources and maximize the expertise inherent in the MMODs.

AMLC: The Way Ahead

As we move forward in our development as a command, we are applying key reforms in five specific areas to address challenges, close gaps, and exploit opportunities.

Visibility and Integration. As a commodity, Class VIII (medical) supply has long struggled with end-to-end visibility and integration into GCSS-Army, the Army's primary enterprise resource planning system. COVID-19 did not identify this issue; it further highlighted the gap and the inability to see ourselves. The good news is that we are attacking the problem and beginning to integrate Class VIII (medical) supply into GCSS-Army, starting with our Army prepositioned stocks, so it can be managed like other commodities and provide better visibility for unit leadership. With the leadership and partnership of US Army Combined Arms Support Command (CASCOM) and CECOM, we will soon integrate Class VIII (medical) supply in GCSS-Army from the tactical level back to the industrial base. This will start in 4th quarter, FY 20, with completion and full integration by the end of FY 22.

Distribution. AMLC is responsible for operational medical logistics; however, medical logistics at stateside military treatment facilities (MTFs) remains under DHA. Nevertheless, we must work together in order to avoid procurement fratricide and inefficiency. We are currently developing a new and revised concept of support that better integrates Class VIII (medical) distribution across the entire enterprise and ensures DHA MTFs remain an alternate source of supply for deploying units that need to access on-hand materiel from these locations.

Planning and Responsiveness. AMLC is improving its demand planning capability by hiring demand planners, determining readiness drivers, and leveraging DLA's medical contingency requirements workflow to provide more accurate information to DLA's medical contingency file, which identifies joint, time-phased, "go-to-war" medical materiel requirements. Our overall purpose is to send an early, accurate demand signal to the industrial base so it can surge, when necessary, to meet the need.

Management and Sustainment. The future of AMLC will see it develop into a life cycle management command (LCMC) with item managers, logistics assistance representatives, national-level purchasing division, and expert senior command representatives that are able to provide direct support at the corps and installation levels. Working collaboratively with program managers and materiel developers at USAMRDC, we must improve Class VIII (medical) materiel management and sustainment plans from inception through divestment or modernization.

Capability and Capacity. Perhaps the biggest lesson learned from COVID-19 is in the way it has challenged our previously held assumptions and thought processes. Traditionally, Army medical logistics planned medical materiel requirements for combat casualties and injuries or illnesses most common for service members in a battlefield environment. Understandably, the type of medical materiel required for trauma (surgical and blood) is very different from that which is required for a pandemic (ventilators and oxygen generating equipment). The burn rate, or speed at which the items are consumed, is also different. In a combat care environment, only the health care providers wear PPE. In a pandemic, the consumption rate for PPE is much higher because non-providers require it.

COVID-19 has taught us to rethink some of the planning factors for replenishment sets. We have been working closely with clinicians and pharmacists to develop new project sets to support rapid, flexible replenishment of single-use parts, such as tubing and valves, on medical devices such as ventilators. This change in thinking will not only help us better support the current pandemic response, but also shape how we sustain future combat operations.

Final Thoughts

While AMLC's transformation was not started by COVID-19, what we have learned from supporting this fight has greatly shaped our reform efforts. Through every challenge, we have sought to find opportunities that generate readiness faster and more efficiently. In many ways, the COVID-19 support mission has provided AMLC with valuable insight of what will be required to meet the size and exponential medical materiel demand in a multi-domain environment, including LSCO.

The contested environment AMLC operates in today is a preview of the future. A huge sports fan, I often distill the challenges of the day to our commanders and staff worldwide by explaining, "there are no lay-ups." Everything is contested on the battlefield. The road to deliver the right effects at the right time is often bumpy and we must be aggressive—but we are on our way.

(This article is available at https://www.army.mil/article/239937/medical_readiness_co vid_19_response_shaping_the_future_of_medical_logistics)

Notes

1. Army Materiel Command (AMC): the primary provider of materiel to the United States Army. The Command's mission includes the research & development of weapons systems as well as maintenance and parts distribution. 陆军器材司令部

2. Army Futures Command (AFC): tasked with driving the Army into the future to ensure the Army and its soldiers overmatch their adversaries in future conflicts. In civilian terms, this means AFC will be focused on the development of new equipment, processes and doctrine to propel the army into the future. AFC leadership is responsible for the Army's research and development (R&D) effort, the Army's future warfare think-tank and modernizing the Army's training and education efforts. 陆军未来司令部

3. United States Army North (USARNORTH): or the Fifth Army (美国第五集团军),

is an Army Service Component Command (ASCC) of the United States Army. It is responsible for homeland defense and defense support of civil authorities as the joint force land component command of United States Northern Command (USNORTHCOM). 美国陆军北方司令部

4. USCENTCOM: United States Central Command, a theater-level Unified Combatant Command of the US Department of Defense, established in 1983. Its area of responsibility includes countries in the Middle East, North Africa, and Central Asia, most notably Afghanistan and Iraq. 美国中央总部

Words and Expressions

1. tactical: *adj.* connected with the particular method you use to achieve something 战术上的；策略上的

2. combatant: *adj.* engaged in or ready for combat 战斗的；好斗的

n. a person or group involved in fighting in a war or battle 战斗人员；战士

3. realign: *v.* to make changes to something in order to adapt it to a new situation 改组；重组

4. stakeholder: *n.* a person or company that is involved in a particular organization, project, system, etc., especially because they have invested money in it 权益相关者

5. calibration: *n.* the act of checking or adjusting (by comparison with a standard) the accuracy of a measuring instrument 标定；校准

6. interoperability： *n.* the ability of a system to work with or use the parts or equipment of another system 互操作性；互用性

7. theater: *n.* the place in which a war or fighting takes place 战场；战区

8. recapitalization: *n.* changing the capital structure of (a corporation) 资本重组

9. collaboration: *n.* the act of working with another person or group of people to create or produce something 合作

10. hone: *v.* to develop and improve something, especially a skill, over a period of time 磨练，训练

11. bolster: *v.* to improve something or make it stronger 改善；加强

12. replenish: *v.* to make something full again by replacing what has been used 补充；重新装满

13. repository: *n.* a place where something is stored in large quantities 仓库；贮藏室；存放处

14. procurement: *n.* the process of obtaining supplies of something, especially for a government or an organization 采购，购买

15. fratricide: *n.* the crime of killing people of your own country or group; a person who is guilty of this crime 杀害同胞行为

16. contingency: *n.* a possibility that must be prepared for; a future emergency 偶发事

件；应急措施

17. orchestrate: *v.* to organize a complicated plan or event very carefully or secretly 精心安排；策划

Exercises

I. Reading Comprehension

A. Directions: Decide whether the following statements are True or False according to the text.

1. AMLC is a direct-report unit to AMC.

2. The new AMLC was formed as a headquarters over four medical logistics subcommands.

3. Today, AMLC serves as the Army's primary medical logistics and sustainment command.

4. AMLC's unit deployment packages (UDPs) included potency and dated items tailored to each medical team's needs.

5. AMLC prepositioned ventilators and ventilator resupply kits at various locations stateside for USCENTCOM.

6. Medical logistics is a lean specialty.

7. The Army sought to decentralize medical logistics with the other sustainment functions inherent within AMC.

8. AMLC collaborated with stakeholders to orchestrate the delivery of medical materiel.

9. Medical logistics at stateside military treatment facilities (MTFs) remains under AMLC.

10. In a combat care environment, only health care providers wear PPE.

B. Directions: Answer the following questions according to your understanding of the text.

1. What are the three medical logistics subcommands under AMLC?

2. What are the four lines of effort within the SSA construct of AMLC to support AMC?

3. Which two states in the US were initially hit hardest by COVID-19?

4. What did the author think was the biggest lesson learned from COVID-19?

5. How did AMLC leverage Army Prepositioned Stocks to provide worldwide support to the pandemic response?

6. Inside AMC, how did integration and synchronization with the other direct reporting units and teammates help AMLC?

7. How does AMLC routinely coordinate with Joint Partners and Key Stakeholders?

8. What are the key reforms of AMLC in five specific areas to address challenges, close gaps, and exploit opportunities?

II. Vocabulary

Directions: Choose the best word or expression from the list given for each blank. Use each word or expression only once and make proper changes when necessary.

stakeholder	contingency	hone	realign
theater	tactical	calibration	combatant

1. He was given _____ command of the operation.

2. I have never suggested that U.N. forces could physically separate the _____ in the region.

3. Following the plant shutdown, New Hampshire Yankee _____ senior management at the plant.

4. The government has said it wants to create a _____ economy in which all members of society feel that they have an interest in its success.

5. Its color _____ is a bit better, although the Galaxy S4 has a more accurate white.

6. We should be prepared for any _____.

7. The Chinese People's Liberation Army has five _____ Commands.

8. Leading companies spend time and money on _____ the skills of senior managers.

III. Topics for Discussion

1. What do you think we can learn from the AMLC response to COVID-19 pandemic in regard to medical logistics?

2. In this article, the author talked about the responses to COVID-19 by AMLC. Please collect relevant information about China's effort to fight COVID-19 and make a comparison between the responses in the two countries.

Text B
Tracking Virus Outbreaks in the Twenty-First Century

Nathan D. Grubaugh

Emerging viruses have the potential to impose substantial mortality, morbidity and economic burdens on human populations. Tracking the spread of infectious diseases to assist in their control has traditionally relied on the analysis of case data gathered as the outbreak proceeds. Here, we describe how many of the key questions in infectious disease epidemiology, from the initial detection and characterization of outbreak viruses, to transmission chain tracking and outbreak mapping, can now be much more accurately addressed using recent advances in virus sequencing and phylogenetics. We highlight the utility of this approach with the hypothetical outbreak of an unknown pathogen, "Disease X", suggested by the World Health Organization to be a potential cause of a future major epidemic. We also outline the requirements and challenges, including the need for flexible platforms that generate sequence data in real time, and for these data to be shared as widely and openly as possible.

Outbreak detection

Most infectious disease outbreaks start with clinicians noticing unusual patterns. Patients may present with patterns of symptoms that are similar to those of more common diseases, but which, after repeated observation and diagnostic testing, may deviate in scale, seasonality or severity. At this very beginning of an outbreak, the most critical task is therefore to identify a causal pathogen. Historically, virus identification has been performed using molecular tools, such as polymerase chain reaction (PCR)[1] and enzyme-linked immunosorbent assay (ELISA)[2], that directly recognize pathogen-derived material, or conventional non-molecular techniques, such as microscopy. The advent of untargeted metagenomic sequencing directly from clinical samples, however, means that we are now on the cusp of being able to detect human viruses in a single step, without a priori knowledge of putative causal pathogens. The major advantage of sequencing-based approaches is the ability to detect novel viruses—such as the initial appearances of SARS2, MERS3 or Lujo virus—or unexpected ones, as exemplified by Ebola virus during the 2013-2016 epidemic in West Africa.

Once an outbreak has been detected and a causal virus identified, several basic questions can immediately be answered about the virus itself, including: (1) whether it is novel or previously known to infect humans; and (2) if we have the diagnostics, vaccines and therapeutics available to fight it. Importantly, the generation of virus genomics data at this stage will provide deeper insights into these questions by uncovering molecular details not possible with conventional tools. Phylogenetics will also provide an additional level of detail, revealing virus origins, evolutionary characteristics and connections to previous outbreaks in the same region, or to transmissions in other regions. Given high enough relatedness to other members of a virus family with well-defined reservoir hosts (for example, old-world arenaviruses), the sequence identification of novel virus species can also be informative about potential reservoirs.

First snapshot of an outbreak

Immediately after a viral outbreak has been identified there exists a "fog-of-war". The extent of the outbreak, the timing and nature of its source, and the contribution of human-to-human transmission will be extremely limited, yet these data are critical to designing effective responses. Genomic epidemiology, if applied quickly and comprehensively, holds the potential to answering these questions.

Transmission chain tracking

Beyond the initial characterization of an outbreak, virus genome sequencing offers enormous potential for determining transmission chains to understand networks of "who-infected-whom". The tracking of transmission chains has long been a standard part of public health responses to outbreaks, providing critical information that can be used to interrupt virus spread and reduce the magnitude of an outbreak. This work has traditionally been performed using interview-based contact tracing, which is labour intensive and limited by the availability and openness of patients for interviews. This approach is particularly challenging during large outbreaks characterized by large numbers of co-occurring transmission chains.

Virus genomic-based approaches can provide much more in-depth information compared to traditional non-sequencing based approaches, as the branching patterns of phylogenetic trees approximately correspond to transmission from one case to the next. Virus genome sequences, for example, were used to reconstruct the spread of foot-and-mouth disease virus in the United Kingdom, including the identification of superspreader events. Genomic data also played a critical role in understanding flare-ups during the West African Ebola outbreak, where phylogenetic analyses showed that most of the flare-ups were linked to persistently infected Ebola survivors, thereby demonstrating sexual transmission of the virus. None of these insights would have been possible without virus genomic data.

The utility of virus genomic data for the inference of transmission chains is dependent on several factors, including: (1) the evolutionary rate of the virus, (2) the length of time between the infections of interest, and (3) the proportion of sampled cases, which together determine the resolution of the genetic signal. Although RNA viruses exhibit remarkably high evolutionary rates, their small genome sizes and short epidemiological generation times often result in, on average, less than one substitution per transmission event. Hence, virus genomics alone often cannot be expected to perfectly reconstruct transmission chains at the level of individual infections. Combined with epidemiological data, however, virus genomics provides a powerful tool for restricting the number of possible transmission scenarios and for supporting novel modes of transmission. In addition, most phylogenetics-based transmission chain analyses have been performed using virus consensus sequences (that is, a single genome per sample/patient that represents the average of the virus population), which may limit resolution. However, as virus infections exhibit diverse intra-host populations (containing intra-host single nucleotide variants, iSNVs), newer methods incorporating viral iSNVs may greatly increase the resolution of transmission chain analyses so long as multiple variants are transmitted between hosts.

Outbreak mapping

As described in the previous sections, genomic epidemiology can be used to detect an outbreak, show its origin and elucidate transmission patterns. Evolutionary inferences from virus genomes, unlike non-sequencing based methods, can also be used to dissect the spatial structure and dynamics of spread, as well as to assess how an epidemic may unfold through time and space.

Uncovering the spatial patterns of virus spread during outbreaks is a key objective that has been transformed by genomic epidemiology. Reconstructing a detailed spatial history of virus spread from the origin of an outbreak is generally a task for phylogeographic methods, which provide location estimates for every ancestral node in a virus phylogeny using simple stochastic (or "random walk") models. Phylogeographic analyses, for example, were used to show how Ebola virus spread across West Africa during the 2013-2016 epidemic. Importantly, virus genome sampling with strong spatiotemporal coverage allowed for the dissection of the entire epidemic into a metapopulation of short- and long-lived transmission chains. Similar analyses were also used to show that multiple introductions were responsible for sustaining the 2016 Zika outbreak in Florida. It is important, however, to appreciate the uncertainty of phylogeographic estimates, and to bear in mind that such analyses may only be capable of elucidating partial pictures of outbreak spread. In addition, sampling biases may severely affect these analyses, although the coalescent and birth-death models mentioned above have been extended to account for aspects of virus population structure, making the analyses more robust to sampling heterogeneity.

Phylogeographic inference methods can also be used to provide insights into the factors driving virus spread. Such analyses are enabled by the integration of virus genomics with diverse meta-data sets and are critically dependent on the timeliness of data generation and open sharing. These approaches were initially introduced to confirm the key role of human air transportation in the global circulation of influenza viruses, but they have also been useful in untangling complex virus transmission dynamics on smaller scales.

Future perspective

Genomic epidemiology promises much to the study and control of infectious disease outbreaks, particularly if viral genomes can be acquired and analysed in real time. The accumulated set of these data—together with the rapid development of sophisticated software packages—will provide a valuable resolve for the mitigation and control of future outbreaks. Ultimately, with sufficient genome sequences from individual viral genera and/or families, it may be possible to categorize viruses by their phylogenetic patterns and utilize this information in epidemic preparedness. For example, as well as considering obvious biological features of viruses such as their genome structure and mode of transmission, it may be possible to group viruses according to a series of evolutionary variables such as rate of evolutionary change, extent of antigenic evolution, frequency of recombination, pattern of geographic spread and population dynamics. This information may then help forecast the evolutionary behaviour of any virus, should it re-emerge in human populations, and assist in the selection of future vaccine strains. This information will also help counter the alarmist claims that emerging viruses will evolve novel phenotypes, such as airborne transmission in the case of Ebola virus, that often accompany any major disease outbreak. It is clear, however, that a more fundamental understanding of the genetic and ecological barriers of virus spillover into human populations is needed to better identify risk factors for disease emergence. Long-term capacity building, partnerships with local communities, and commitments to long-term investments on these fronts will go a long way towards better enabling the global community to effectively and rapidly deal with future emerging outbreaks.

(This article is excepted from "Tracking Virus Outbreaks in the Twenty-First Century" published in *Nature Microbiology,* PMID: 30546099)

Notes

1. polymerase chain reaction (PCR): a fast and inexpensive technique used to "amplify"–copy–small segments of DNA. Because significant amounts of a sample of DNA are necessary for molecular and genetic analyses, studies of isolated pieces of DNA are nearly impossible without PCR amplification. Often heralded as one of the most important scientific advances in molecular biology, PCR revolutionized the study of DNA to such an extent that its creator, Kary B. Mullis, was awarded the Nobel Prize for Chemistry in 1993. 聚合酶链式反应

2. enzyme-linked immunosorbent assay (ELISA): an immunological assay commonly used to measure antibodies, antigens, proteins and glycoproteins in biological samples. Some examples include: diagnosis of HIV infection, pregnancy tests, and measurement of cytokines or soluble receptors in cell supernatant or serum. 酶联免疫吸附测定法

Words and Expressions

1. assay: *v./n.* the testing of metals and chemicals for quality, often to see how pure they are 试验；化验含量测定

2. flare-up: *n.* a sudden painful attack, especially after a period without any problems or pain 突发

3. phenotype: *n.* the set of characteristics of a living thing, resulting from its combination of genes and the effect of its environment 表型

4. untangle: *v.* to make something that is complicated or confusing easier to deal with or understand 整理；理清

5. putative: *adj.* believed to be the person or thing mentioned 认定的，假定的

6. spatiotemporal: *adj.* of, relating to, or existing in both space and time 时空的

7. coalescent: *adj.* coming together as a recognizable whole or entity 合并的；接合的

Medical Vocabulary

genomics: 基因组学
polymerase: 聚合酶
metagenomics: 宏基因组学，元基因组学
phylogenetics: 种系遗传学
metagenomic: 宏基因组的
arenaviruses: 沙粒病毒

nucleotide: 核苷酸

Exercise

Critical Thinking

Please summarize how the recent advances in virus sequencing and phylogenetics can be used to facilitate infectious disease epidemiology in the four aspects of initial detection, characterization of outbreak viruses, transmission chain tracking and outbreak mapping.

Supplementary Reading

For more information on Biosafety and Emergency Response, please go to the following websites:

1. https://www.cdc.gov/outbreaks/index.html

2. https://www.canada.ca/en/public-health/services/canadian-biosafety-standards-guidelines/handbook-second-edition/chapter-16-20.html

3. https://www.sciencedirect.com/science/article/pii/S2588933818300189

Unit Eight　Combat and Operational Stress Control

Text A
Getting inside Their Heads

First came the casualties—the grim tally of military dead and wounded. Then, as the wars in Afghanistan and Iraq continued, came post-traumatic stress disorder (PTSD)[1] and traumatic brain injury (TBI)[2] among the troops who came home.

Now the US military is coping with a high-profile incidence of psychological and behavioral problems among troops—from drug addiction, major depression, and suicide to spousal abuse and other violence, rising divorce rates, crime, heavy drinking, and maltreatment of children. And the situation is getting new attention from military medical personnel, top defense officials, veterans' groups, and Congress.

Last year six soldiers from units at Fort Carson, Colorado, were accused of killing eight people over the previous 12 months. The case set off a crash investigation to find what prompted the shooting spree and has made Fort Carson an icon, underscoring the need to tackle the increased behavioral problems among service veterans more effectively. The report, issued in July, said the effects of exposure to combat had been a factor.

A new study by the RAND Corporation[3] estimates that some 18.5 percent of service members returning from Afghanistan and Iraq screen positive for PTSD or depression and says that 19.5 percent have experienced a major or minor traumatic brain injury—together affecting almost one-third of the two million who have been deployed to the war zones.

More broadly, a new study by physicians at the Veterans' Administration (VA)[4] medical center in San Francisco, published in the September 2009 issue of the *American Journal of Public Health*, confirms that more than one-third of the veterans who entered the VA system after serving in Iraq and Afghanistan have been diagnosed with mental health problems. With psychological and behavioral disorders included, the figure topped 40 percent.

1. Linked to Deployments?

To many Americans the reason for the new surge seems obvious. With today's urban warfare and insurgencies, the intensity of the fighting is pronounced. And some troops have been redeployed for two, three, or even four tours.

Critics contend that the stress produced by these deployments—both among the Soldiers and Marines who actually are in combat and among those outside the war zones, who must work harder and often longer to keep the rest of their services operating—has begun to take its toll. The current "dwell-time"—the period troops are permitted back in the States before they deploy again—is only a year.

"What you're really talking about is a stressed-out force," says Retired Air Force Lieutenant General Charles H. Roadman II, a former Surgeon General of the Air Force who has been an adviser to DOD on medical problems affecting troops who have served in combat zones. "This type of warfare is more stressful than what we're used to thinking about. You're actually in combat all day every day."

2. A High Priority

The mental health problem has become acute enough that top military and civilian leaders now openly acknowledge it and have begun taking steps to deal with it. Defense Secretary Robert Gates says that "Other than winning the wars we are in, my highest priority is providing the best possible care for those who are wounded in combat"—including those suffering from psychological and behavioral problems.

The services say they are beginning to screen more of the troops returning from Afghanistan and Iraq. All four branches have set up programs designed to detect psychological and behavioral problems sooner and begin treating them early on. They've established "warrior transition" units to provide injured service members treatment and support.

They also are moving to permit troops more dwell-time between deployments to help them adjust more fully to stateside life—and take a rest from their combat tensions—before they have to go back to the war zone. In some cases, Soldiers or Marines have had barely a few months before having to return to combat—not enough, psychologists say, to make an adequate adjustment.

In a potentially far-reaching step, DOD has established six Defense Centers of Excellence for Psychological Health and Traumatic Brain Injury that will draw on military, VA, and civilian efforts to study and treat psychological disorders. The Army has just launched a $50 million study on suicide and mental health—the largest the military has ever undertaken—that is expected to delve into the causes of the current problems and how to treat them.

3. Shortage of Care-Givers

One major difficulty is that the services don't have enough trained mental health personnel to deal with the surge of cases. Although the Pentagon moved quickly to deploy medical personnel to forward-deployed field hospitals at the start of both wars, it wasn't prepared for either the length of the deployments or the number of troops the two operations would require, says the University of Maryland's David Segal.

A Pentagon Task Force on Mental Health concluded in 2007 that the military's "current complement of mental health professionals is woefully inadequate." And House legislation introduced last year reported that approximately 40 percent of the billets for licensed clinical psychologists in the Army are vacant, and other mental health professions, including psychiatry and clinical social work, also report shortages.

Moreover, Iraq and Afghanistan Veterans of America (IAVA), a New York-based veterans' advocacy group, says mental health support for troops in Iraq actually is declining, with the ratio of behavioral health workers to troops in those combat zones falling to one for every 734 in 2007, from one for every 387 in 2004. And getting a referral to a psychiatrist or psychologist in the Army or Marine Corps takes far longer than it should.

The services have been pushing to expand their medical staffs, but there still are shortages in some categories. DOD figures show that in 2008 the services had 308 psychiatrists on active duty—about 4.5 percent fewer than authorized—and 584 psychologists, or about 14 percent under strength. And the authorizations themselves don't necessarily reflect actual needs.

Both VCS (Veterans for Common Sense)[5] and IAVA have urged Congress to increase the number of mental health professionals and begin providing mandatory face-to-face psychological examinations for troops before they leave for combat zones and when they return.

4. Treatment is Improving

Uncertainty about cause and effect doesn't mean that the services can't treat psychological and behavioral problems. Even the most severe critics concede that the military has improved markedly in handling such cases. Many consider the armed forces to be the cutting edge in identification and treatment of such illnesses, and, more recently, a pioneer in efforts to reduce the problem of stigma, which infects the civilian world as well.

Dr. Robert Ursano, who heads the psychiatry department at the Uniformed Services University of the Health Sciences, says one of the key tasks confronting military medicine over the next few months is to survey the plethora of mental health programs that have been established in recent years, weed out those that are overlapping or aren't working, and then build up those that are producing results. "It's adaptive design," he says. "As soon as information is obtained, we will feed that back to the military so they will implement it."

But the efforts have only begun to expand. "Our challenge at this point is to do a full-court press on the medical front," General Sutton (the Defense Centers of Excellence) says—and to do it as rapidly as possible. Time is not our friend.

(This article is excerpted from *Proceedings*, September/2009)

Notes

1. post-traumatic stress disorder (PTSD): a mental condition in which a person suffers severe anxiety and depression after a very frightening or shocking experience, such as an accident or a war. Post-traumatic stress disorder (PTSD) is a mental health condition that's triggered by a terrifying event—either experiencing it or witnessing it. 创伤后应激障碍

2. traumatic brain injury (TBI): often referred to as TBI, is most often an acute event similar to other injuries. That is where the similarity between traumatic brain injury and other injuries ends. 创伤性脑损伤

3. RAND Corporation: It is a research organization that develops solutions to public policy challenges to help make communities throughout the world safer and more secure, healthier and more prosperous. 兰德公司

4. Veterans' Administration (VA): It is a government-run military veteran benefit system with Cabinet-level status. （美国）退伍军人福利管理局

5. Veterans for Common Sense (VCS): founded in 2002, a non-profit organization dedicated to advocacy on behalf of United States veterans who continue to serve their country by protecting the rights and interests of fellow citizen 退伍军人共识组织

Words and Expressions

1. casualty: *n.* someone injured or killed or captured or missing in a military engagement 伤亡人员

2. traumatic: *adj.* of or relating to a physical injury or wound to the body 创伤的

3. disorder: *n.* condition in which there is a disturbance of normal functioning 混乱

4. billet: *n.* lodging for military personnel (especially in a private home) 部队临时营地（尤指民宅）

5. weed out: to remove unwanted elements 清除；淘汰

6. delve into: to search for something inside a bag, container, etc.（在手提包、容器等中）翻找

7. accuse of: to bring an accusation against; to level a charge against 谴责，控告

8. cope with: to deal with or fulfill 处理，应付

9. underscore: *v.* to give extra weight to (a communication); to emphasize 强调

10. surge: *n.* rise or heave upward under the influence of a natural force such as a wave 汹涌；蜂拥而来

11. pronounced: *adj.* strongly marked; easily noticeable 显著的；断然的

12. take its toll: to harm or damage somebody or something, especially in a gradual way 造成损失，造成伤害

13. concede: *v.* to admit; to make a clean breast of; to give over 承认；让步

14. cutting- edge: *adj.* the leading position in any movement or field 领先的，尖端的

15. confront: *v.* to deal with (something unpleasant); to head on 面对；遭遇

Medical Vocabulary

psychological and behavioral problems: 心理和行为疾病
major depression: 重度抑郁症
heavy drinking: 酗酒

psychological and behavioral disorders：心理和行为障碍

licensed clinical psychologist：执业临床心理学家

dwell-time：轮休期

a full-court press on the medical front：在医疗界全面推行

warrior transition unit：官兵调适单位

Defense Centers of Excellence：国防卓越中心

Pentagon Task Force on Mental Health：五角大楼精神健康工作组

Exercises

I. Reading Comprehension

A. Directions: Decide whether the following statements are True or False according to the text.

1. The high-profile incidence of psychological and behavioral problems among US troops is getting new attention from military medical personnel, top defense officials, veterans' groups, and Congress.

2. According to the report issued in July, exposure to battles had been a factor in the shooting spree at Fort Carson, Colorado.

3. Two million service veterans who have been deployed to the war zones have been affected by PTSD, depression and TBI.

4. Based on the study published in *American Journal of Public Health*, more than one-third of the veterans in the VA system after serving in Iraq and Afghanistan had been diagnosed with mental health problems. With psychosocial and behavioral disorders included, the number increased by 40 percent.

5. The current "dwell-time" for the troops is merely a year.

6. As critics contend, the stress produced by intense deployments also influences the troops outside the war zones, because they have to work harder and often longer to keep the rest of their services operating.

7. It can be inferred from Part 1 that the US troops are mentally and physically exhausted.

8. Considering the length of the deployments and the number of troops the two war operations would require, the Pentagon moved quickly to deploy medical personnel to forward-deployed field hospitals.

9. According to House legislation introduced in 2008, the vacancy for clinical psychologists in the Army is about 40 percent.

10. In reality, it takes far longer than it should if one needs to see a psychiatrist or psychologist in the Army or Marine Corps.

B. Directions: Answer the following questions according to your understanding of the text.

1. What are the typical psychological and behavioral problems among US troops that the

US military is coping with?

2. What makes Fort Carson an "icon"?

3. Who are the victims of PTSD and TBI?

4. According to Lieutenant General Charles H. Roadman II, why is this type of warfare more stressful than what we're used to thinking about?

5. What is Department of Defense (DOD)'s highest priority?

6. How did the ratio of behavioral health workers to troops in Iraqi combat zones fall between 2004 and 2007?

7. Based on Para 16, what should be the authorized number of psychiatrists on active duty in the services? How about the authorized number of psychologists?

8. As urged by VCS and IAVA, when should mandatory face-to-face psychological examinations be taken for US troops?

9. What will be one key task confronting military medicine over the next few months according to the text?

II. Vocabulary

Directions: Choose the best word or expression from the list given for each blank. Use each word or expression only once and make proper changes when necessary.

| concede | pronounced | weed out | surge | shortage |
| cutting-edge | delve into | underscore | confront | cope with |

1. What we are planning is _____ technology never seen in Australia before.

2. Moving your body on a regular basis is a helpful way of _____ chronic stress. Even a daily 20-minute walk makes a difference.

3. China won't _____ an inch on South China Sea and Taiwan.

4. The problems _____ the new government were enormous.

5. The company _____ the incompetent people.

6. Flood waters _____ into their homes.

7. Because I was eager to _____ that novel further, I decided to write about it for my term paper.

8. Many healthcare facilities experienced staffing _____ during COVID-19.

9. The energy crisis _____ the need to increase fuel efficiency.

10. He walked with a _____ limp.

III. Topics for Discussion

1. What problems are facing US troops from Afghanistan and Iraq? What are the causes of these problems?

2. What measures do the services and DOD take to deal with the current problem?

Text B
A Healthy Soldier is a Ready Soldier

R. Scott Dingle

There is an African proverb that states, "It takes a village ..." This maxim also holds true for the holistic approach required for soldiers who are ready, lethal and able to meet the Army's needs.

Initiatives from the US Army Futures Command's Soldier Lethality Cross-Functional Team recognize the importance of a holistic approach to soldier lethality. The emphasis is on building the physical supremacy, cognitive dominance and emotional resilience required for a soldier to excel in a multidomain operation. This requires a whole-of-Army approach to understand the human dimension of warfare.

While many appreciate the historic mission Army Medicine has fulfilled to "conserve the fighting strength," the story is more complex. New initiatives from across the Department of the Army are expanding the approach to health and readiness to ensure that the soldier remains the most prized weapon system on today's and tomorrow's battlefield. From an enterprise perspective, the Military Health System can be viewed as an employer-based provider and payer of care, one of the largest in the nation, caring for 9.4 million beneficiaries. For Army Medicine, that employer happens to be an expeditionary Army where readiness of the force is the most critical population health outcome.

Therefore, unlike CEOs of a civilian hospital, a military medical treatment facility commander is required to also serve as an installation's director of health services. Over the past decade, as Army Medicine has transitioned from a health care system to a system for health and readiness, the roles of the director of health services have dramatically shifted and expanded. Army Medicine is no longer the traditional "find it and fix it" civilian medical clinic, but rather a community focused on:

1) Prediction, preemption and prevention.

2) Early identification and intervention.

3) Evaluation and treatment.

4) Rehabilitation and reintegration after injury and disease.

These changes empower a medical treatment facility to act as both a health care network and an agent of public health. It can expand health outside brick-and-mortar facilities and operate where people live, love and labor to best translate health care delivery into readiness through physical, cognitive and emotional health. This model of approaching health from the installation level is population-focused, emphasizes health care collaboration, and focuses on improving the main population outcome for beneficiaries.

This article will outline and highlight the non-health care delivery roles and responsibilities of the director of health services to build a medically ready force and improve community and installation health at the operational level and the tactical level.

Soldier Support

The most powerful weapon system in the Army will always be the soldier. Spurred by 2017 National Defense Authorization Act(NDAA)[1] legislative changes, Army medical treatment facilities have effected installation-level changes to ensure soldiers are physically, mentally and emotionally ready to "Fight Tonight."

One of the main health issues that impacts readiness is musculoskeletal injuries. In 2017, active-duty soldiers experienced 1,821 new injuries for every 1,000 person-years, affecting over half of all soldiers each year, according to the Army's "2018 Health of the Force" report. The impact of injuries is staggering and typically results in about 10 million limited-duty days per year. To address this, the director of health services works with US Army Forces Command partners to support and coordinate early identification efforts, and to profile review boards, physical training curriculums and other programs. These efforts, coupled with physical therapists embedded within the brigade, have dramatically decreased the injury burden on readiness.

The "2018 Health of the Force" report also says 15% of soldiers have a behavioral health disorder. To address these conditions, the director of health services must appoint a senior behavioral health officer as the installation director of psychological health to leverage all available behavioral health capabilities, providing collaborative, full-spectrum services. The installation director of psychological health leads the Behavioral Health Working Group within the Community Ready and Resilient Council (CR2C), synchronizing a broad array of spiritual-, community-, mental health- and family-oriented programs to form a continuum of preventive inpatient or outpatient care.

Integrated behavioral health consultants within primary care medical homes provide routine behavioral health support for outpatient medicine clinics, including smoking cessation, sleep hygiene, non-medication pain management and healthy living. The Army's practice of embedding behavioral health staff far forward has also improved medical readiness outcomes. Pre- and post-deployment transitions are known periods of stress on soldiers and their families.

Because of the close relationships with organic unit behavioral health and chaplain assets, embedded teams are able to ensure early comprehensive services are provided to soldiers and families in need. This provides a stable environment for mission focus and, ultimately, readiness. Early detection and treatment resulted in a significant decrease in the number of inpatient behavioral health bed days utilized by service members.

The director of health services programs supports the unique readiness challenges of female soldiers, who make up 15% of the active-duty force. In addition to Army Medicine's mandate to provide high-quality care for pregnant women, additional programs ensure female soldiers are physically, cognitively and emotionally ready after delivering a baby.

One example is Pregnancy Postpartum Physical Training (P3T)[2], an Army-unique, standardized, holistic, physical training and educational program to help soldiers maintain fitness during pregnancy and postpartum recovery. Nearly 70% of P3T participants surveyed affirmed the program's efficacy in helping them pass elements of their fitness tests, and 29% said it influenced them to remain in the Army, according to the "2016 Health of the Force" report.

Another program, called Centering Pregnancy, groups women with similar delivery dates whose extended families are not close enough geographically to support them. Also, recognizing the critical role of nutrition on development and readiness, the director of health services at Fort Riley, Kansas, invited a representative from the Women, Infants and Children program into the post hospital to help ensure optimal nutrition during and after pregnancy.

Army Medicine is also moving from isolated programs that address individual medical concerns to holistic programs that incorporate a range of them. For example, if a soldier has previously struggled with weight gain and body composition, programs such as Fit for Performance and Army Wellness Centers are in place to augment medical treatment to help ensure a fit and ready soldier returns to the force.

Similar programs exist for soldiers who become ill and struggle with passing Army physical fitness tests. The Move to Health program builds the patient-provider relationship and synchronizes treatment with many of the Army Medicine, garrison and community resources addressing exercise and nutrition, family and community, and behavioral health resources to improve soldier rehabilitation and reintegration after illness or injury.

Army Medicine's Performance Triad promotes daily habits for improved sleep, activity and nutrition. A 2016 National Training Center study found that company-sized elements that did not integrate sleep-management strategies failed to receive a rating of above average (a rating of 4 out of 5) for sleep habits—a significant threat to cognitive dominance and emotional resilience. A variety of data-driven strategies, ranging from techniques for sleep banking to reverse-cycle training to targeting the use of chemical interventions such as caffeine, are provided to leaders to improve the sleep quantity and quality of their units. Nutrition and activity targets and tips are also emphasized to provide reasonable and effective strategies for improvement. The Performance Triad has a significant preventive health impact and strongly improves readiness.

Leader Support

Leader support and engagement is key to successfully improving overall and individual health readiness. At Schofield Barracks[3], Hawaii, the senior commanding general's quarterly executive CR2C was tri-chaired by the garrison commander and the director of spiritual health with the director of health services to identify and address the health readiness needs of the post. These needs are then communicated with CR2C working groups to fully synchronize available installation resources behind the Army's best practices, allowing quicker adoption of readiness-building practices.

The 25th Infantry Division at the Schofield Barracks CR2C implemented a "flipped classroom" concept for its council, in which the data-driven CR2C slides were viewed before the meeting, allowing the council to become a discussion forum for health-readiness challenges, gaps, requirements and solutions.

"The flipped CR2C has allowed subject-matter experts from the physical, behavioral, spiritual, social and family working groups to better understand the needs of the command teams that they support," said Col. Steve Dawson, US Army Hawaii garrison commander. "The true value of the flipped CR2C is the dialogue that occurs between the brigade commanders, senior leaders and working group subject-matter experts. It is during this dialogue that the commanders share the wisdom that they gleaned from their health of the force data."

Army Medicine has also been leading the charge to translate data to wisdom for division, brigade, battalion and company command teams by creating dashboards and tools to better understand medical readiness and inform decision-making by unit leaders. The new e-profile facilitates leader-provider conversations, enhances profile review board processes and helps ensure data can inform readiness decisions.

According to Whitfield East's 2013 monograph, the most important aspect of unit physical training is to awaken the warrior spirit each morning. Programs in which physical therapists, occupational therapists and dietitians work with line leadership to enhance unit physical training can be successful.

Community, Installation Support

Fundamentally, readiness starts at home. To help create cultural change aligned with Army priorities on readiness, communities of excellence are developed to build a culture that embraces a holistic approach to building soldier and family readiness. Across an installation, the health care system supports Soldier and Family Readiness Groups, Senior Spouse Groups, school programs and other outreach efforts that ultimately facilitate readiness. At Schofield Barracks, for example, a nonprofit organization called Warriors at Ease was integrated into unit physical training, recovery programs at the medical treatment facility and community-based events to integrate yoga into training and promote overall health and wellness. This program quickly grew in popularity across the installation.

At the installation level, the medical treatment facility, along with members across the installation, supports the creation of Healthy Army Communities. It has three tools to assess the physical environment and policies on installations related to nutrition, physical activity and tobacco.

The medical treatment facility's dietitian supports the implementation of DOD's Go for Green program[4] to improve healthy options at dining facilities and vending machines to promote readiness. All these tools apply choice architecture and build on scientific principles to assess and improve the environments where people live, work and play, increasing visibility and ability to make the healthy choice the easy choice.

Fundamentally, Army Medicine exists to save lives on the battlefield and generate readiness for an expeditionary Army to fight and win our nation's wars. As the director of health services, the medical treatment facility commander exists to enable human performance optimization and build a more lethal and resilient force by focusing on maintaining, restoring and improving the physical, cognitive and emotional readiness of our soldiers.

(The full article is available at https://www.ausa.org/articles/healthy-soldier-ready-soldier)

Notes

1. National Defense Authorization Act (NDAA)： Each year, NDAA authorizes funding levels and provides authorities for the US military and other critical defense priorities, ensuring troops have the training, equipment, and resources they need to carry out their missions. 《国防授权法》

2. Pregnancy Postpartum Physical Training (P3T): a standardized physical training and education program designed to enable pregnant and postpartum soldiers to maintain fitness, organized as a mandatory, weekly workout for all pregnant and postpartum, active-duty soldiers 孕妇产后运动训练

3. Schofield Barracks: home to the 25th Infantry Division, Schofield Barracks is nestled at the foot of the Waianae mountain range on the island of Oahu in Hawaii. The 17,725-acre Schofield Barracks site was established in 1908 to provide a base for the Army's mobile defense of Pearl Harbor and the entire island. 斯科菲尔德兵营

4. Go for Green program: the US Army's dining facility nutrition education program. Go for Green is a nutritional recognition labeling system providing the soldier with a quick assessment of the nutritional value of menu offerings and food products in the dining facility. The menu offerings and food items are labeled green (eat often), amber (eat occasionally), and red (eat rarely) based on the impact the food can have on a soldier's performance. 绿色食品计划

Words and Expressions

1. lethality: *n.* the quality or condition of causing death 杀伤力；致命性；毁坏性

2. beneficiary: *n.* a person who gains as a result of something 受益者；受惠人

3. expeditionary: *adj.* sent on or designed for military operations abroad 远征的；探险的

4. preemption: *n.* the action of preempting, as the use of military force in a preemptive attack 先发制人

5. brick-and-mortar: *adj.* located or serving consumers in a physical facility as distinct from providing remote, especially online, services 实体的

6. spur: *v.* to incite or stimulate 激励；促进

7. staggering: *adj.* so great, shocking or surprising that it is difficult to believe 令人震惊的；令人难以相信的

8. brigade: *n.* a large group of soldiers that forms a unit of an army 旅

9. synchronize: *v.* to happen at the same time or to move at the same speed as something 同步；同时发生

10. array: *n.* a group or collection of things or people, often one that is large or impressive 大群；大量

11. cessation: *n.* the stopping of something 停止；中断

12. chaplain: *n.* a priest or other Christian minister who is responsible for the religious needs of people in a prison, hospital, etc. or in the armed forces（监狱、医院、军队等的）牧师；特遣牧师

13. garrison: *n.* a group of soldiers living in a town or fort to defend it 卫戍部队；守备部队；

14. triad: *n.* a group of three related people or things 三人组合；三位一体

Exercise

Critical Thinking

According to this article, what kinds of health services can improve the physical, cognitive and emotional readiness of our soldiers? What's the situation in Chinese army? Please search the information and have a discussion with your partner.

Supplementary Reading

For more information on Combat and Operational Stress Control, please go to the following websites:

1. https://irp.fas.org/doddir/army/fm4-02-51.pdf

2. https://www.workplacementalhealth.org/Case-Studies/Naval-Center-for-Combat-Operational-Stress-Control

3. https://www.armyupress.army.mil/Portals/7/military-review/Archives/English/SO-21/hoyt-combat-operational-stress/hoyt.pdf

Unit Nine　Precision Medicine

Text A
Precision Medicine[1]: What Barriers Remain?

Chris Lo

Precision medicine holds immense promise as a facilitator of more targeted therapies and a healthier society. But with adoption proving slow out of the gate, what are the challenges that remain before the full potential of personalised healthcare can be reached?

The importance of the individual has been widely established in medicine since time immemorial. The well-worn adage that physicians should "treat the patient, not the disease" has been around since the 19th century, and the awareness of that message is far older than that. Even Hippocrates, the "father of Western medicine" who treated patients in the fifth century BC, stressed the importance of treating each patient as an individual.

"For the sweet [medicines] do not benefit everyone, nor do the astringent ones, nor are all patients able to drink the same things," Hippocrates wrote.

Hippocrates might have tailored his rudimentary treatments based on the patient's age, physique and other easily observable factors, but personalized medicine in the 21st century offers the promise of therapies customised based on the study of what truly makes us unique: our DNA.

The promise of personalized medicine

Advancements in genomics, proteomics, data analysis and other fields—both medical and technical—are gradually facilitating the development of laser-focused drugs, as well as the ability to predict people's personal risk factors for particular diseases and how individual responses to various treatments might differ.

After years of anticipation, there is now evidence that governments around the world have clocked the importance of personalised medicine and are driving efforts to build the genetic data sets and biobanks that are required to push the science forward. Former US President Barack Obama launched the Precision Medicine Initiative[2] to great fanfare in 2015; the scheme has since evolved into the All of Us Research Programme[3], which aims to gather health data from more than a million US volunteer-citizens to unlock new insights.

In the UK, the 100,000 Genomes Project reached its goal of sequencing 100,000 whole genomes from 85,000 NHS[4] patients with cancer or rare diseases. Genomics England has noted that so far, analysis of this data has revealed "actionable findings" in around one in four rare disease patients, while about 50% of cancer cases suggest the potential for a therapy or clinical trial.

"You can match a blood transfusion to a blood type—that was an important discovery," said Obama at the launch of the Precision Medicine Initiative, summarising the broad appeal of personalised therapies and diagnostics. "What if matching a cancer cure to our genetic code was just as easy, just as standard? What if figuring out the right dose of medicine was as simple as taking our temperature?"

Early days: slow progress on clinical adoption

The stage might be set for personalised healthcare to dramatically transform public health, but few in the medical field would deny that the world is hardly ready yet. Transitioning from the traditional one-cure-fits-all treatment model to new processes that leverage patients' genetics, lifestyles and environmental risk factors is an immense task that presents challenges in both the laboratory and the clinic.

Oncology is, by a landslide, the field that has been most impacted by developments in precision medicine; around 90% of the top-marketed precision treatments approved in 2018 were cancer therapies, while other therapeutic areas have lagged far behind. The majority of approved precision medicines in oncology achieve something of a halfway house between the old way and the new—they fall short of being tailored to a specific individual, but they allow for more detailed stratification of patients by the oncogenic mutations of their tumours, which may be driving cancer cell survival and growth.

Common examples of these mutations are HER-2 in certain breast and stomach cancers, BRAF in melanoma and EGFR in lung cancer. High expression of these proteins at cancer sites can be targeted by precision treatments, such as Roche[5]'s monoclonal antibody Herceptin (trastuzumab) for HER-2, Genentech[6]'s BRAF inhibitor Zelboraf (vemurafenib), and Roche's EGFR inhibitor Tagrisso (osimertinib). Regulators such as the US Food and Drug Administration (FDA) and the European Medicines Agency (EMA) are also increasingly approving "tumour-agnostic" treatments—the first and most famous of which is Merck[7]'s immunotherapy Keytruda (pembrolizumab)—which target specific biomarkers regardless of tumour location.

But despite the availability of a growing menu of personalised cancer treatments, actually matching patients up to the right therapy can be difficult. According to a survey of US acute care organisations conducted by Definitive Healthcare and published in December 2019, just over 20% had established precision medicine programmes. Investment in genomic testing is vital to quickly get patients on the best treatment course, but financial and operational barriers remain.

The foremost among these is the cost associated with genomic sequencing and the use of companion diagnostic devices, cited by 28% of Definitive Healthcare's respondents as the biggest challenge for already-established precision medicine schemes. Lack of expertise is another obstacle, as many physicians may struggle to accurately interpret test results without specialist assistance—another major cost driver for clinics and hospital departments trying to build pathology teams that are up-to-date with the newest tests. A 2018 survey of 160 oncologists by Cardinal Health found that 60% of physicians who don't use genomic tests avoid them because of the difficulty of interpreting the data.

Precision medicine barriers in drug development

In clinical research and development, too, there are growing pains associated with moving the pharmaceutical pipeline towards drugs targeting smaller patient sub-groups. Again, cost is a central issue—companion diagnostics don't come cheap, finding and validating biomarkers to guide targeted therapies is a lengthy task, and analysing vast amounts of data often requires new teams with specialised knowledge.

The expense of incorporating a host of new processes into innovative trial designs—not to mention the cost of manufacturing cell and gene therapies—obviously has an impact on the list price of personalised drugs that win approval. This is most clearly seen in the eye-watering prices of some of the world's first truly individualised cancer treatments, chimeric antigen receptor T-cell (CAR-T) therapies.

Treatments such as Novartis[8]'s Kymriah and Gilead[9]'s Yescarta remove T-cells from the patient's blood, modify them to target tumour cell antigens and then infuse them back into the blood stream. These therapies have achieved impressive results in rare and advanced cancers, but cost upwards of $400,000 per patient, limiting their reimbursement options among both private and public payers. Promising advances in CAR-T manufacturing and potential "off-the-shelf" T-cell production could help bring these costs down in the years to come, but for now the problem remains.

As for the broader clinical trial eco-system, these studies have been historically set up to assess a drug candidate's safety and efficacy in an increasingly large segment of the patient population, building evidence towards the regulatory approval process. Bringing a personalized medicine through the clinical development process is a new paradigm in a number of ways; as well as the aforementioned cost drivers, there can be an extra enrolment burden to identify and recruit patients—this is already a common cause of trial failure, but it's all the more difficult when you're looking to access a small patient sub-group with the appropriate biological profile.

Regulatory uncertainty

The difficulty of providing sufficient evidence of safety and efficacy can also present issues where current regulations struggle to accommodate new innovations in personalised medicine. Smaller trial designs present statistical problems in terms of understanding a drug's definitive risk-benefit profile, and while some "personalized" applications can be discovered as part of larger trials that fail to meet their endpoints outside of a select patient group with particular biomarkers, many current regulations don't accept post hoc analysis and would require an entirely new trial.

"Personalised medicine developers desire better guidance on how best to design a successful clinical trial for a personalised therapy, because absent guidance, they risk presenting suboptimal evidence regarding stratification options," reads a 2017 study on personalised medicine barriers, published in the *Journal of Law and Biosciences*. "Designing clinical trials for differently responding subgroups (for example, biomarker-positive and biomarker-negative groups) requires additional time and resources. Companies are reluctant to make this investment without a commensurate increase in the certainty of regulatory approval."

The increasing use of surrogate endpoints, conditional approvals and real-world data is helping to address these issues, but they're not yet an ideal solution. Conditional approvals rely on very careful post-marketing observation and analysis, while the value of surrogate endpoints has been questioned, adding to the tension between accelerating approvals and ensuring patient safety.

The ultimate benefits of creating more personalised treatments are clear, and their advantages for human health could, in the long-term, be matched by their economic returns. After all, quickly treating patients with the right therapy for them—or, even better, using knowledge of a patient's genetic risk profile to prevent illness in the first place—would be a huge financial gain for overburdened health systems.

Today's costs are gradually falling, as NIH[10] data on DNA sequencing costs demonstrate. But there is still a long way to go before we can wave goodbye to the blanket drug development that has dominated modern pharma for decades, even in the advanced field of oncology, let alone other therapeutic areas. Only a sustained and holistic push—from regulators, drug developers, clinicians, governments and others—will be enough to bring us over the line.

(The full article is available at https://www.pharmaceutical-technology.com/features/precision-medicine-2020/)

Notes

1. precision medicine: a medical model that proposes the customization of healthcare, with medical decisions, treatments, practices, or products being tailored to a subgroup of patients, instead of a one-drug-fits-all model 精准医疗

2. the Precision Medicine Initiative: a research program created in 2015 during the tenure of Barack Obama with $130 million in funding that aims to make advances in tailoring medical care to the individual 精准医疗计划

3. the All of Us Research Program me: previously known as the Precision Medicine Initiative Cohort Program. The mission of AoU is to accelerate health and medical breakthroughs, enabling individualized prevention, treatment and care. 全民健康研究计划

4. NHS: (the National Health Service) the British system that provides free medical treatment for everyone, and is paid for by taxes 国民医疗服务体系（英国的免费医疗制度）

5. Roche: a Swiss multinational healthcare company that operates worldwide under two divisions: Pharmaceuticals and Diagnostics 瑞士罗氏（制药企业）

6. Genentech: an American pioneering research-driven biotechnology company which became a subsidiary of Roche in 2009 美国基因工程技术公司，简称基因泰克

7. Merck: a German multinational science and technology company founded in 1668, the world's oldest operating chemical and pharmaceutical company, as well as one of the largest pharmaceutical companies in the world 德国默克公司

8. Novartis: a Swiss multinational pharmaceutical company based in Basel, Switzerland. It is one of the largest pharmaceutical companies in the world. 诺华公司（瑞士制药公司）

9. Gilead: an American biopharmaceutical company headquartered in Foster City, California, that focuses on researching and developing antiviral drugs used in the treatment of HIV, hepatitis B, hepatitis C, and influenza 美国吉利德科学公司

10. NIH: The National Institutes of Health is the primary agency of the United States government responsible for biomedical and public health research. It was founded in the late 1880s and is now part of the United States Department of Health and Human Services. 美国国立卫生研究院

Words and Expressions

1. facilitator: *n.* something that helps a process to take place 辅助器

2. immemorial: *adj.* starting longer ago than people can remember, or than written history shows 年代久远的

3. adage: *n.* a well-known phrase that says something wise about human experience 格言，谚语

4. astringent: *adj.* having a sharp acid taste 味涩的

5. rudimentary: *adj.* simple and basic 基本的，初步的

6. clock: *v.* to notice someone or something 注意到

7. fanfare: *n.* a lot of activity, advertising, or discussion relating to an event 大张旗鼓的宣传

8. leverage: *v.* to spread or use resources, ideas etc. 充分利用

9. stratification: *n.* the division of something into different layers 分层

10. agnostic: *adj.* unknown, unknowable 不可知的

11. upwards: *adv.* more than a particular amount, time etc.（数量、时间等）……以上

12. reimburse: *v.* to pay back to somebody (money that he has spent, lost, etc.); to refund something 补偿，报销

13. off-the-shelf: *adj.* already made and available in shops rather than being designed especially for a customer 现成的

14. paradigm: *n.* a model or example that shows how something works or is produced 模型，范式

15. post hoc: happening after the event 事后的

16. commensurate: *adj.* matching something in size, quality, or length of time 与……相当的，相称的

17. surrogate: *adj.* a surrogate person or thing is one that takes the place of someone or something else 替代的，代理的

18. holistic: *adj.* considering a person or thing as a whole, rather than as separate parts 整体的，全面的

Medical Vocabulary

oncogenic: 致瘤的；瘤原性的

melanoma: 黑素瘤

trastuzumab: 曲妥珠单抗

vemurafenib: 威罗非尼

osimertinib: 奥西替尼

pembrolizumab: 派姆单抗

chimeric: 嵌合的

Exercises

I. Reading Comprehension

A. Directions: Decide whether the following statements are True or False according to the text.

1. Personalized medicine remains a mixed blessing for major governments in the world, leaving them hesitant to devote serious money into it.

2. The British Genomes Project not only attained the goal of genome sequencing, but also obtained valuable information for future therapy.

3. Compared with the public, medical professionals are more confident that we are ready for embracing personalized healthcare.

4. Few approved precision medicines in oncology are customized for specific individuals.

5. CAR-T therapies with daunting prices are a vivid manifestion of the financial barrier to personalized drugs.

6. Recruiting a small patient sub-group to test personalized treatments is comparatively easier than enrolling a large group of the patient population.

7. Smaller personalized trials are accepted as part of larger ones under many current regulations.

8. Despite its benefits and advantages, personalized medicine has not reaped economic

gains.

9. In the field of oncology, traditional paradigm of drug development will continue to dominate for a long time.

10. Success in precision medicine ultimately depends on drug developers and medical professionals.

B. Directions: Answer the following questions according to your understanding of the text.

1. According to Definitive Healthcare, what is the greatest challenge to the precision medicine programs already in place?

2. In what way is the lack of expertise an obstacle?

3. What are the obstacles to development of drugs targeting smaller patient sub-groups?

4. What is the medical procedure involved in CAR-T treatments?

5. What statistical problems are likely to be found in smaller trial designs?

6. Why do personalized medicine developers need better guidance?

7. Why does the author argue that surrogate endpoints and conditional approvals are not yet an ideal solution?

8. How does the author view the prospects of personalized treatments?

II. Vocabulary

Directions: Choose the best word or expression from the list given for each blank. Use each word or expression only once and make proper changes when necessary.

reimburse	commensurate	holistic	paradigm
leverage	facilitate	rudimentary	stratification

1. It was a _____ device and it wasn't until 1921 in Berkeley, California, when the official polygraph machine for lie detecting was invented.

2. That's when we changed the _____ of medicine from one of secrecy and hiding to one that is fully open and engaged.

3. Japanese real wages have not yet increased _____ with the wealth of Japan.

4. I'm really interested in seeing how I can _____ the software to do something that hasn't been done with it before.

5. In sociology, social _____ is the hierarchical arrangement of social classes, castes and strata within a society.

6. The great cultural impact of printing was that it _____ the growth of national languages.

7. Families of people who died in the aftermath of the storm are eligible to have some of their funeral expenses _____ by the US government.

8. The Food and Agriculture Organization is calling for a _____ approach to meet the growing disease threat.

III. Topics for Discussion

1. What are the benefits promised by personalized medicine?

2. Describe the progress of precision medicine in oncology.

3. Summarize all the barriers that remain in the field of precision medicine.

Text B
A Longitudinal Big Data Approach for Precision Health

Sophia M. S. Rose

Abstract

Precision health relies on the ability to assess disease risk at an individual level, detect early preclinical conditions and initiate preventive strategies. Recent technological advances in omics and wearable monitoring enable deep molecular and physiological profiling and may provide important tools for precision health. We explored the ability of deep longitudinal profiling to make health-related discoveries, identify clinically relevant molecular pathways and affect behavior in a prospective longitudinal cohort (n = 109) enriched for risk of type 2 diabetes mellitus. The cohort underwent integrative personalized omics profiling from samples collected quarterly for up to 8 years (median 2.8 years) using clinical measures and emerging technologies including genome, immunome, transcriptome, proteome, metabolome, microbiome and wearable monitoring. We discovered more than 67 clinically actionable health discoveries and identified multiple molecular pathways associated with metabolic, cardiovascular and oncologic pathophysiology. We developed prediction models for insulin resistance by using omics measurements, illustrating their potential to replace burdensome tests. Finally, study participation led the majority of participants to implement diet and exercise changes. Altogether, we conclude that deep longitudinal profiling can lead to actionable health discoveries and provide relevant information for precision health.

Precision health and medicine are entering a new era in which wearable sensors, omics technologies and computational methods have the potential to improve health and lead to mechanistic discoveries. Emerging technologies such as longitudinal multi-omics profiling combined with clinical measures can comprehensively assess health and identify deviations from healthy baselines that may improve disease risk prediction and early detection. Connecting longitudinal multi-omics profiling with clinical assessment is also important for developing a new taxonomy of disease on the basis of molecular measures.

Despite this promise, few studies have leveraged emerging technologies and longitudinal profiling to manage health and identify disease markers. Previous efforts included our study of a single individual in which longitudinal multi-omics profiling over 14 months captured the individual's transition to diabetes on a deep molecular level. A recent study of 108 individuals followed for 9 months using various omic technologies revealed several health-related findings. A cross-sectional study used genome sequencing, metabolomics and advanced imaging to identify individuals at risk for age-related chronic disease. These studies had limited sample size, lacked meaningful longitudinal profiling or performed only limited analysis of health information. We have also demonstrated the use of wearable devices to detect infections and identify early glucose dysregulation and population-based studies evaluating arrythmia detection are underway.

In the present study, we longitudinally profiled 109 participants at risk for diabetes mellitus (DM), performing quarterly clinical laboratory tests and multi-omics assessments. In addition, individuals underwent exercise testing, enhanced cardiovascular imaging and physiological testing, wearable sensor monitoring and completed various surveys.

The study objectives were three-fold. We first evaluated the usefulness of emerging technologies in combination with standard and enhanced clinical tests to detect diseases early. We then characterized multi-omics associations with clinical pathophysiologies including glucose and insulin dysregulation, inflammation and cardiovascular risk; we also evaluated the ability of multi-omics measures to predict insulin resistance and response to glucose load. Last, we examined how participation affected health habits.

Results

Summary of research design and cohort. A 109-person cohort enriched for individuals at risk for DM underwent quarterly longitudinal profiling for up to 8 years (median 2.8 years) using standard and enhanced clinical measures and emerging assays. Emerging tests included molecular profiling of the genome, gene expression (transcriptome), proteins (proteome), immune proteins (immunome), small molecules (metabolome) and gut microbes (microbiome), and wearable monitoring including continuous glucose monitoring (CGM). Our study was designed to capture transitions from normoglycemic to pre-DM and from pre-DM to DM. Thus, in addition to standard measures such as fasting plasma glucose (FPG, reflects steady-state glucose metabolism) and glycated hemoglobin (HbA1C, reflects 3-month average glucose), enhanced measures included the oral glucose tolerance test (OGTT, reflects response to glucose load) with insulin secretion assessment (beta-cell function) and the modified insulin suppression test measuring steady-state plasma glucose (SSPG, a measure of peripheral insulin resistance). We also performed enhanced cardiovascular profiling including vascular ultrasound, echocardiography, cardiopulmonary exercise testing and cardiovascular disease protein markers. Technical details are provided in the methods and our integrated Human Microbiome Project (iHMP) paper. The study was approved by the Stanford University Institutional Review Board (IRB 23602) and all participants consented.

The mean age of integrated personalized omics profiling (iPOP)[1] participants at initial enrollment was 53.4±9.2 years old. Genetic ancestry analysis (n=72) using the 1,000 Genomes Project (1,000GP) data shows that individuals mapped to expected ancestral populations.

Over the study course, we found over 67 major clinically actionable health discoveries spanning metabolism, cardiovascular disease, oncology and hematology, and infectious disease. We demonstrated ways in which longitudinal multi-omics measures can be used to advance precision health, including by illuminating biological pathways underlying standard measures, predicting burdensome physiological measurements and enabling exploration of mechanisms of disease onset.

Discussion

Our study found that combining untargeted multi-omics and physiological longitudinal profiling with targeted profiling of metabolic and cardiovascular risk led to actionable health discoveries and meaningful physiological insights building on our previous work. Our targeted profiling approach enabled us to connect longitudinal profiling of glucose metabolism with multi-omics profiling facilitating the precision medicine goal of defining diseases on the basis of molecular mechanisms and pathophysiology. The untargeted longitudinal big data approach led to a number of discoveries in other areas such as cardiology, oncology, hematology and infectious disease, indicating that broad profiling is valuable for disease detection in many different areas. We capitalized on the depth of longitudinal profiling to identify deregulated molecules and pathways associated with the transition from health to disease.

The study informed more than half the participants of their pre-DM and DM status, dyslipidemia and hypertension, which led many to institute diet and physical activity lifestyle changes. Our enhanced clinical assays including OGTT, beta-cell function assessment, insulin resistance and CGM in combination with standard clinical tests (FPG and HbA1C) improved characterization of pre-DM and DM status. The in-depth physiological profiling identified individual mechanisms of glucose dysregulation that has important implications for implementation of personalized treatments. Our findings are consistent with a recent study that found that treatments based on the current classification are not well tailored to mechanistic subtypes and proposed five subtypes of adult onset DM. Deeper molecular understanding of progression to DM and its characteristics in the individual may help tailor therapy to its underlying pathophysiology and will probably identify additional subtypes and also inform stratification of CVD risk. The superiority of using multi-omics data for SSPG prediction compared to standard measures illustrates the value of multi-omics data to help provide a molecular taxonomy of disease, as well as replace expensive burdensome tests for insulin resistance with a simple blood test. Microbiome measures were also a good predictor of SSPG when combined with clinical measures and SSPG inversely correlated with Shannon diversity further demonstrating the intricate relationship between gut microbes and insulin resistance consistent with our multi-omics study of weight gain.

Although the majority of our exome sequencing findings were in the oncologic realm, several important metabolic exome findings were found including a MODY mutation with implications for medication management, an *RBM20* mutation related to dilated cardiomyopathy and numerous pharmacogenomic variants that have important health implications. Furthermore, two participants experienced vascular events, unaware of relevant pharmacogenomics information that could have suggested alternative treatments. Thus, we expect complex genetic risk assessment such as the information learned in this study to be incorporated into risk management and tailored treatment of disease.

Imaging plays a central role in precision health initiatives, enabling the early detection of oncological and systemic disease. In our study, imaging helped detect dilated cardiomyopathy (in the patient with *RBM20* mutation), early stage atherosclerotic disease and a case of asymptomatic lymphoma. Wearable sensors are emerging as a transformative technology for precision health and medicine and heart rate monitoring led to the diagnosis of atrial fibrillation, sleep apnea and detection of Lyme disease in participants. Large population-based initiatives such as "myHeart counts" are evaluating the potential of wearable heart sensors to detect subclinical atrial fibrillation and electrocardiographic monitoring is now available in consumer wearable devices. Our findings also suggest a role for CGM in diabetes prevention by identifying unrecognized glucose dysregulation, and enabling the individual to optimize their diet on the basis of personalized glycemic responses.

Our multi-omics analysis also provided important insights into ASCVD risk, highlighting the importance of systemic inflammation. Although our study was not powered for outcome analysis, all five participants with incident cardiovascular events had subclinical inflammation. Furthermore, correlation network analysis highlighted the role of monocytes, HGF, IL-2, MCP-3 and interferon-gamma cytokines including MIG and IP10 and other molecules in cardiovascular health. These analytes are involved in inflammation and are emerging in the context of ASCVD.

Untargeted longitudinal outlier analysis of the period leading up to the diagnosis of lymphoma illustrates the importance of longitudinal multi-omics analysis for biomarker and pathway discoveries. We identified potential critical biomarkers (for example, MIG) and changes in the microbiome up to 1 year before diagnosis demonstrating the power of monitoring molecules longitudinally to detect deviations from the healthy baseline. Outlier biomarkers at time of diagnosis illustrated deregulated pathways related to inflammation, cell proliferation and cell migration that shed light on underlying dysregulated biological mechanisms associated with the disease. Further work will be needed to streamline the investigation of untargeted discoveries in precision medicine research. Given the need for early biomarkers for cancer detection, longitudinal multi-omics analyses represent an important tool for meeting this need. In addition to individual molecule monitoring, omics profiles provide the opportunity to detect outliers relative to a matched-healthy population. Clinical outlier analysis identified one participant with MGUS where early diagnosis with follow-up can increase survival time in individuals who progress to an associated malignancy. While some omics outlier profiles could be clearly connected to an underlying health condition, the case of the participant with significant RNA-seq outliers illustrates the challenges of interpreting the clinical relevance of outlier analysis results with emerging measures. While precision medicine approaches have the potential for unnecessary anxiety and overtesting, we did not observe this in our population.

In the rapidly evolving field of precision medicine, this study should be assessed in the context of methodological considerations. Our cohort comprised highly educated volunteers, and therefore probably had a self-selection bias. Although this may affect the generalizability of our findings for behavioral changes, it is less likely to affect the underlying biological associations of multi-omics with glucose measures. A study strength is its ethnic diversity, which is greater than that in other longitudinal multi-omics studies. In sum, we demonstrate the feasibility of a longitudinal precision health and medicine approach that builds on sound molecular and physiological phenotyping. We show that in-depth physiological and multi-omics characterizations are likely to further refine risk stratification. The intensive longitudinal study design demonstrates how a small longitudinal cohort can yield important health and discovery findings. In the future, it will be possible to design personalized testing programs on the basis of individual disease risk and longitudinal marker trajectories as well as evaluate the cost-value of these approaches for individuals and health care systems.

(The full text is available at https://www.nature.com/articles/s41591-019-0414-6)

Notes

1. integrated personalized omics profiling (iPOP): a longitudinal study of approximately 100 individuals meant to help lay a foundation for precision personalized medicine through the unprecedented deep biochemical profiling of generally healthy individuals. It is designed to understand what "healthy" biochemical and physiological profiles look like at a personal level and what happens when people become ill. The study was designed and is performed at Stanford University. 个体化多组学整合分析

Words and Expressions

1. profiling: *n.* the activity of collecting information about someone or something 分析

2. longitudinal: *adj.* involving the repeated observation or examination of a set of subjects over time with respect to one or more study variables 纵向的

3. illuminate: *v.* to make clear; to help to explain 阐明

4. capitalize (on): *v.* to gain by turning something to advantage 利用

5. tailor: *v.* to make or adapt something for a special purpose 量身打造

6. inverse: *adj.* reversed in position, direction or relation 相反的，成反比的

7. intricate: *adj.* made up of many small parts put together in a complex way, and therefore difficult to follow or understand 错综复杂的

8. deviation: *n.* difference between a numerical value and a norm or average 偏差

9. shed light on: to make something clearer 使某事显得非常清楚；使人了解某事

10. trajectory: *n.* the events that happen during a period of time, which often lead to a particular aim or result 发展轨迹

Medical Vocabulary

omics: 组学

immunome: 免疫组

transcriptome: 转录组

proteome: 蛋白质组

metabolome: 代谢组

microbiome: 微生物组

insulin resistance: 胰岛素抵抗

taxonomy: 生物分类学

arrythmia: 心律失常

normoglycemic: 血糖正常的

fasting plasma glucose: 空腹血糖

glycated hemoglobin: 糖化血红蛋白

dyslipidemia: 血脂异常

exome: 外显子组

dilated cardiomyopathy: 扩张型心肌病

pharmacogenomics: 药物基因组学

atherosclerotic: 动脉粥样硬化的

lymphoma: 淋巴瘤

atrial fibrillation: 房颤

sleep apnea: 睡眠呼吸暂停

monocyte: 单核细胞

Exercise

Critical Thinking

This study is one of the leading investigations in the rapidly evolving field of precision medicine. Please discuss with your partner what you know about precision medicine, what latest advances have been reported in literature, and how these developments may affect individuals and health care systems.

Supplementary Reading

For more information on Precision Medicine, please go to the following websites:

1. https://www.fda.gov/medical-devices/in-vitro-diagnostics/precision-medicine

2. https://www.cdc.gov/genomics/about/precision_med.htm

3. https://www.nih.gov/about-nih/what-we-do/nih-turning-discovery-into-health/promise-precision-medicine

Unit Ten   Smart Military Medical Technology

Text A
Why Super Soldiers May Soon be a Nightmare Turned Reality

Alex Hollings

While Captain America[1] was first introduced to audience way back in March of 1941, the Marvel Cinematic Universe[2]'s depiction of the scrawny kid turned brawny hero in *Captain America: The First Avenger*[3] brought the concept out of the '40s and into the modern consciousness. Since then, there's been no shortage of articles comparing the titular hero to ongoing efforts to pull the best possible performance out of the human form, but how practical are these efforts really? It turns out, they're increasingly practical.

Of course, it's important to remember that not every scientific effort to improve human performance is inherently related to the military. While Captain America benefitted from defense research in his own transition into the peak of human capability, today's pharmaceutical conglomerates and university-backed researchers are making significant strides toward improving human performance in the private sector. In a truly all-encompassing "super soldier" effort, the research, treatments, and even body modifications found in these other endeavors would almost certainly play a vital role—and to be clear, that's the way the Pentagon[4] would probably prefer.

In recent years, the Defense Department has placed an increased emphasis on leveraging "off the shelf" technology that's already been developed in the private sector. This approach offers massive cost-savings over the traditional method of soliciting proposals and awarding contracts for research and development, as well as a vastly expedited delivery. The more off-the-shelf components a new defense program leverages, the faster it can go from theory to fruition. This mindset works for rifles and night-vision goggles, but could also feasibly work for the sort of medical treatments and technologies the Pentagon would need to successfully start fielding super soldiers.

So, let's take a look at some defense and private sector programs that could very feasibly help usher in the age of super heroes on the battlefield.

Engineered blood could offer huge performance boosts

The human body was designed for a pretty rigorous lifestyle, but an engineering design for a not-too-distant artificial red blood cell could very literally give future super-soldiers a significant leg up over the competition. These artificial red blood cells, called respirocytes, would give their users the ability to hold their breath for extended periods of time and offer a massive jump in cardiovascular endurance.

These tiny machines would be made up of just three parts: rotors to absorb and release oxygen, rotors to absorb and release carbon dioxide, and rotors to absorb and release glucose. In effect, the respirocytes would do the same job as red blood cells, just far better than nature could permit. The concept is based on the work of Robert Freitas, a nanotechnology researcher at the Institute for Molecular Manufacturing[5], and would offer the user the ability to "hold their breath at the bottom of a swimming pool for four hours, or let someone sprint at top speed for at least 15 minutes without stopping to breathe."

Being able to hold your breath for hours would obviously come in handy for Special Operators approaching from the shore, and the added endurance offered by these super-cells would come in handy in just about every combat environment on the planet.

Night vision could be injected straight into your eyes

Today, American service members in theater often operate using night-vision goggles (NVGs), but these systems offer some real drawbacks. The standard NVGs issued to troops on the ground offer very little peripheral vision and even less depth perception, making them tough to adjust to and increasing the risk of dangerous operations like driving at speed or engaging opponents under fire. Special Operations units often have better night vision options, but with civilian equivalents recently hitting the market at around $40,000 per pair, these more capable goggles are too cost-prohibitive for broad distribution... but what if we didn't need them anymore?

In a recent study from the University of Massachusetts Medical School in Worcester, MA, mice were trained to navigate a maze by following triangular signs they'd come across along their way. Then, with the lights off, they'd let the mice try again with exactly the results you'd expect: They couldn't find their way in the dark. Then, scientists injected mice with nanoparticles that convert infrared light to visible light directly into their eyeballs. The result was a newfound ability to see in the dark that lasted for around 10 weeks and seemed to offer no negative side effects.

Turning thoughts into firepower on the battlefield

For all of Captain America's talents, he's never managed to pull off reading minds or telekinesis, but these sorts of skills may become standard issue in the years ahead. A decade ago, the Defense Advanced Research Projects Agency (DARPA)[6] was already experimenting with helmets that would allow for "silent talk." The goal was to read a user's pre-speech brainwaves and convert them into transmittable data. The recipient's system would receive and translate that data into audible or visual cues in the recipient's headset.

This would allow soldiers on the battlefield to communicate while maintaining total silence, but the uses for this sort of tech extend well beyond whispering secrets into your squad leader's ear. In 2018, DARPA announced that an individual equipped with their experimental brain-computer interface had successfully controlled a constellation of three different types of simulated aircraft simultaneously with her mind.

This sort of tech could lead to fighter pilots who can control their AI-equipped drone wingmen from programs like the Air Force's Skyborg[7] or Boeing's Loyal Wingman[8] programs seamlessly through thought. In the future, the same tech could be leveraged for other drone and semi-autonomous air, sea, and ground platforms—allowing our war fighters to bring their own heavy reinforcements with them, or even to control robotic exoskeletons they wear into the fight.

Getting yoked like Cap

The most important facet of Captain America's super soldier serum was its ability to transform him physically from an underweight weakling into a heavyweight champ, but just how feasible is that?

Steroids and other performance-enhancing drugs have been around for some time, and let there be no mistake, there have already been instances of these sorts of drugs being used for military applications. However, using anabolic steroids requires a carefully controlled treatment plan that includes medications that can offset your body's own efforts to produce higher levels of estrogen in order to offset the added testosterone in your system. Failing to adequately manage hormones can lead to serious health issues, including the sorts we all grew up hearing about among needle-pushing bodybuilders.

According to E. Paul Zehr, the director for the Centre for Biomedical Research at the University of Victoria, hormone and gene therapies that are already used to treat, cure, or supplement patients could eventually be leveraged to turn an ordinary soldier into something a bit more super.

Zehr posits that similar treatments could be used to push a person's physical capabilities to the outside limits of human potential. He cites practices found in livestock, like removing myostatin genes from Belgian Blue Cattle to allow them to develop massive amounts of muscle, as a practical demonstration of what could be done to human subjects. He believes that combining these treatments with a clinically developed training regimen could result in human beings that are as much as 30% stronger than the strongest gym-rat in your squad bay.

For now, it seems all but certain that future battlefields will see super soldiers of one form or another—be they genetically, biologically, or technologically modified (or perhaps all three). Being first doesn't always mean best, and like every arms race before it, there's sure to be a few surprises along the way.

(The full article is available at https://www.sandboxx.us/blog/why-super-soldiers-may-soon-be-a-nightmare-turned-reality/)

Notes

1. Captain America: a superhero who appears in comic books published by Marvel Comics. The character first appeared in *Captain America Comics* (cover-dated March 1941). 美国队长

2. the Marvel Cinematic Universe: MCU, an American media franchise and shared universe that is centered on a series of superhero films, independently produced by Marvel Studios and based on characters that appear in American comic books published by Marvel Comics 漫威电影宇宙

3. *Captain America: The First Avenger*: a 2011 American superhero film based on the Marvel Comics character Captain America《美国队长：复仇者先锋》

4. the Pentagon: the headquarters building of the United States Department of Defense. As a symbol of the US military, the phrase "the Pentagon" is also often used as a metonym or synecdoche for the Department of Defense and its leadership. 五角大楼（也指代美国国防部）

5. the Institute for Molecular Manufacturing: a nonprofit molecular nanotechnology research organization 分子制造研究所

6. the Defense Advanced Research Projects Agency (DARPA): a research and development agency of the United States Department of Defense responsible for the development of emerging technologies for use by the military 美国国防部高级研究计划局

7. Skyborg: the United States Air Force Vanguard program developing unmanned combat aerial vehicles intended to accompany a manned fighter aircraft 美国空军"天空堡"项目

8. Loyal Wingman: also known as the Boeing Airpower Teaming System (ATS), is a stealth, multirole, unmanned aerial vehicle in development by Boeing Australia for the Royal Australian Air Force designed as a force multiplier aircraft capable of flying alongside manned aircraft for support and performing autonomous missions independently using artificial intelligence 波音"忠诚僚机项目"

Words and Expressions

1. scrawny: *adj.* not having much flesh 瘦的；皮包骨的

2. brawny: *adj.* very large and strong 身体强壮的；肌肉发达的

3. titular: *adj.* held as the result of having a title 有称号的

4. inherent: *adj.* existing as a natural or permanent feature or quality of somebody/something 内在的；固有的

5. conglomerate: *n.* large corporation formed by merging several different firms（通过合并若干企业而组建的）大公司

6. stride: *n.* rapid progress 进展

7. all-encompassing: *adj.* including everything 包罗万象的

8. gym rat: someone who spends a lot of time exercising at the gym 健身达人

9. solicit: *v.* to ask for (eg money, help, votes) earnestly; to try to obtain 恳求（某人）给予（钱、帮助等）；设法获得

10. expedite: *v.* to hasten or speed up 加快；加速

11. mindset: *n.* someone's general attitude, and the way in which he thinks about things and makes decisions 思维模式

12. rigorous: *adj.* very thorough and strict 严格的，严密的

13. literally: *adv.* actually, exactly 确实地；真正地

14. a leg up: an advantage over others 优势

15. sprint: *v.* to run a short distance at full speed 短距离全速奔跑

16. equivalent: *n.* thing, amount or word that is the same 对应物

17. prohibitive: *adj.* (of prices, etc.) so high that one cannot afford to buy（指价格等）高得买不起的

18. cue: *n.* an action or event that is a signal for something else to happen 提示；信号

19. constellation: *n.* a group of associated or similar people or things 一群，一组

20. simulate: *v.* to reproduce (certain conditions) by means of a model, etc., for study or training purposes（用模型等）模拟（某环境）

21. drone: *n.* an uncrewed aircraft or ship guided by remote control or onboard computers 无人机

22. seamlessly: *adv.* done or made so smoothly that you cannot tell where one thing stops and another begins 无缝地

23. yoke: *v.* to unite or form a bond between 使结合或联合

24. champ: *n.* the same as a champion 冠军

25. offset: *v.* to compensate for or balance something 补偿或抵消

26. posit: *v.* to suggest or assume as a fact 假定；假设

27. regimen: *n.* a special plan of food, exercise etc. that is intended to improve your health 养生之道，生活制度

Medical Vocabulary

respirocyte: 呼吸细胞

rotor: 转子

glucose: 葡萄糖

peripheral vision: 周边视野

telekinesis: 心灵感应

steroid: 类固醇

anabolic: 合成代谢的

estrogen: 雌激素

testosterone: 睾丸激素

myostatin: 肌肉生长抑制素

Exercises

I. Reading Comprehension

A. Directions: Decide whether the following statements are True or False according to the text.

1. The scientific advance to enhance human performance can be attributed to the combined efforts of military and private sectors.

2. Off-the-shelf technology works better for speeding up delivery than for cutting down cost.

3. The super cells known as respirocytes can be applicable to almost all combat environments.

4. American soldiers equipped with standard night-vision goggles may find themselves at risk during dangerous night operations.

5. In the experiment conducted by the University of Massachusetts Medical School, the mice injected with nanoparticles suffered irreversible side effects.

6. Being able to read minds is not only a trait that makes Captain America a superhero, but also a potential secret weapon to arm future American troops.

7. The experiment on mind control with brain-computer interface has yet to produce promising results.

8. Creation of super soldiers by hormone therapy requires rigorous treatment plans.

9. Zehr believes what has been done to Belgian Blue Cattle may pave the way for future experiments on human subjects.

10. In the race for super soldiers, it pays to be the first to roll out prototypes.

B. Directions: Answer the following questions according to your understanding of the text.

1. How does the Pentagon view the progress in enhancing human performance in the private sector?

2. What are the benefits of off-the-shelf technology?

3. How can respirocytes give super soldiers a leg up over their opponents?

4. What were the findings of the investigation on mice from the University of Massachusetts Medical School?

5. How did DARPA's helmets make "silent talk" possible?

6. In what ways would DARPA's brain-computer interface help in future warfare?

7. What notes of caution should we bear in mind when using steroids and other performance-enhancing drugs? And why?

8. According to Zehr, to what extent is it possible to push a person's physical

capabilities?

II. Vocabulary

Directions: Choose the best word or expression from the list given for each blank. Use each word or expression only once and make proper changes when necessary.

inherent	offset	regimen	simulate
cue	solicit	rigorous	equivalent

1. How has being _____ curious impacted your career?

2. His party has just suffered the _____ of a near-fatal heart attack.

3. Some diets are more sensible than others, but any _____ that promises swift and dramatic results will doom most followers to failure.

4. According to official documents, government officials _____ bribes several times from local businessmen in exchange for the awarding of state contracts.

5. The expressions on people's faces give us visual _____ about their feelings.

6. The transfusion treatment will need to undergo _____ testing to determine if it makes a difference.

7. US airports are seeking $10 billion in government assistance to _____ losses spurred by this pandemic.

8. Using computational modeling, they then _____ what sort of blasts could have produced those movements.

III. Topics for Discussion

1. Summarize the potential performance-enhancing benefits of each of the four super-hero programs mentioned in the text.

2. Which of the four super-hero programs is most likely to become a reality? Why do you think so?

3. In your opinion, what other aspects of human potentials can be tapped in order to create super soldiers?

Text B
An Epidermal Patch for the Simultaneous Monitoring of Haemodynamic and Metabolic Biomarkers

Juliane R. Sempionatto

Abstract

Monitoring the effects of daily activities on the physiological responses of the body calls for wearable devices that can simultaneously track metabolic and haemodynamic parameters. Here we describe a non-invasive skin-worn device for the simultaneous monitoring of blood pressure and heart rate via ultrasonic transducers and of multiple biomarkers via electrochemical sensors. We optimized the integrated device so that it provides mechanical resiliency and flexibility while conforming to curved skin surfaces, and to ensure reliable sensing of glucose in interstitial fluid and of lactate, caffeine and alcohol in sweat, without crosstalk between the individual sensors. In human volunteers, the device captured physiological effects of food intake and exercise, in particular the production of glucose after food digestion, the consumption of glucose via glycolysis, and increases in blood pressure and heart rate compensating for oxygen depletion and lactate generation. Continuous and simultaneous acoustic and electrochemical sensing via integrated wearable devices should enrich the understanding of the body's response to daily activities, and could facilitate the early prediction of abnormal physiological changes.

Intertwined with concepts of telehealth[1], the Internet of medical things, and precision medicine, wearable sensors offer features to actively and remotely monitor physiological parameters. Wearable sensors can generate data continuously without causing any discomfort or interruptions to daily activity, thus enhancing the self-monitoring compliance of the wearer and improving the quality of patient care. Monitoring of single physical parameters, such as the electrocardiogram and blood pressure (BP), as well as biochemical parameters, such as glucose, using non-invasive wearable sensors has been reported. The importance of integrating multiple sensors on a single device has been demonstrated, where multiple chemical sensors were integrated into a single wrist band. Following this pioneering work, sensor integration is now shifting towards the combination of different sensor modalities. Recent efforts have led to the integration of physical and chemical sensors into a single wearable device—such as combining electrocardiography electrodes with lactate or glucose sensors to monitor the cardiovascular performance, metabolism, electrolyte balance, or the body temperature of an athlete. However, to the best of our knowledge, the in-depth study of the correlation of cardiovascular parameters, particularly BP, with biomarker levels using an integrated hybrid wearable sensor remains unexplored.

Heart rate (HR) and BP, two of the most important vital signs, can dynamically and directly reflect the physiological status of the body. These cardiovascular parameters can be affected by fluctuations of various biomarker concentrations originating from activities such as movement, stress or the intake of food, drinks and drugs that can lead to sudden and sometimes lethal alterations. Parallel BP-chemical sensing could thus have clinical value, especially for people with underlying health conditions—such as the elderly or individuals who are obese, or those affected by diabetes and cardiovascular diseases—as their physiological response to normal day-to-day activities might differ from healthy individuals. Furthermore, the prevention, diagnosis and treatment of many diseases can benefit greatly from simultaneous monitoring of cardiovascular parameters and biomarker levels. These include acute and deadly septic shock, which commonly involves a sudden drop in BP accompanied by rapidly increasing blood-lactate levels, and hypoglycaemia- or hyperglycaemia-induced hypotension or hypertension, which increase the risk of stroke, cardiac diseases, retinopathy and nephropathy in patients with diabetes. Tracking of metabolites and haemodynamic parameters using the same device can increase the self-monitoring compliance of a patient, as it simplifies the complex process of using multiple devices for measuring these parameters, thereby circumstantially preventing dangerous cardiac events and saving lives. The combination of transdisciplinary sensing modalities into a single miniaturized skin-conformal wearable device can yield additional advantages. For example, critically ill and premature infants need continuous monitoring of various dangerous conditions, ranging from hypoglycaemia and sepsis-like infection to open-heart surgery, where BP and the level of lactate or glucose need to be monitored continuously. The neonate-monitoring systems available at present require the application of multiple, often invasive, sensors coupled to bulky instruments on their tiny bodies that pose severe injury risks and barriers to parent-baby bonding. By integrating different sensing modalities on a single flexible, skin-worn tattoo-like patch, vulnerable patients—from neonates to the elderly—can leverage their monitoring device with minimal discomfort or obtrusiveness. The recent global pandemic has also highlighted the urgent need for remote self-monitoring devices, with particular attention to the management of high BP and diabetes, which are major factors in the death of patients with coronavirus disease 2019. A comprehensive cardiovascular/biomarker self-monitoring system would enhance the self-awareness of users to their health conditions and alert them as well as their caregivers to the occurrence of abnormal physiological changes.

Here we present a conformal, stretchable and integrated wearable sensor that can monitor BP, HR and the levels of glucose, lactate, caffeine and alcohol towards dynamic and comprehensive health self-monitoring. We use ultrasonic transducers to monitor BP and HR, and electrochemical sensors to measure the levels of biomarkers. Through strategic material selection, layout design and fabrication engineering, we integrated rigid and soft sensor components, namely customized piezoelectric lead zirconate titanate (PZT) ultrasound transducers and printed polymer composites via an innovative solvent-soldering process into a single wearable conformal sensor with high mechanical resiliency and an absence of sensor crosstalk. Such rational design overcomes engineering challenges related to the integration of different sensing modalities and materials to allow real-time monitoring of cardiovascular parameters and biomarker levels in connection to parallel sampling of the interstitial fluid (ISF) and sweat biofluids. The resulting epidermal hybrid device can emit ultrasonic pulses and sense echoes from arteries while stimulating sweat and extracting ISF through iontophoresis (IP), thereby allowing parallel measurements of BP and HR along with multiple biomarkers in these biofluids. We carried out on-body trials on several human volunteers undergoing various activities and stimuli (exercise and the intake of alcohol, food and caffeine; Fig. 10-1d). The correlations between metabolic variations and haemodynamic activities under these stimuli were monitored and evaluated. The improved sensor assembly process, leveraging the styrene-ethylene-butylene-styrene block copolymer (SEBS)-based stretchable materials, allowed a fast and reliable fabrication of the stretchable and conformal epidermal sensor for acoustic and electrochemical sensing. Such a device offers comprehensive tracking of the effect of daily activities and stimuli on the physiological status of the user, and enables the collection of previously unavailable data towards understanding the body response to such stimuli while addressing the critical post-pandemic needs for remote telemetric patient monitoring.

The multimodal sensing wearable patch is depicted in Fig. 10-1a. SEBS was used as the stretchable and conformal substrate to support the electrodes and connections printed with customized inks (Fig. 10-1e). The stretchable substrate and inks allow the high conformity, flexibility (Fig. 10-1f(i)) and stretchability (Fig. 10-1f(ii)) required for wearable devices. The BP sensor consists of an array of eight piezoelectric transducers that are aligned with the carotid artery on application to the neck to obtain optimal ultrasonic signals. During sensing, the piezoelectric transducers were activated with electrical pulses, transmitting ultrasound beams to the artery, and the time of flight of the echoes from the anterior and the posterior walls of the artery was analysed to gauge the dilation and contraction of the arteries (Fig.10-1c,h). The optimal BP signal can be selected from the eight transducers with the best alignment to the artery and hence the highest signal quality, thus ensuring reliable BP sensing during movement, when the patch may undergo some displacement. Chemical sensing was realized through non-invasive sweat stimulation (via transdermal pilocarpine delivery) at the IP anode, along with ISF extraction at the IP cathode. Lactate, alcohol and caffeine were monitored only in sweat, whereas glucose was monitored only in the ISF. Chronoamperometry (CA) was used for the electrochemical detection of the hydrogen peroxide product of the glucose oxidase, lactate oxidase and alcohol oxidase enzymatic reactions, whereas differential pulse voltammetry (DPV) was used for the detection of caffeine. The analytical performance of each chemical sensor is shown in Fig. 10-1g.

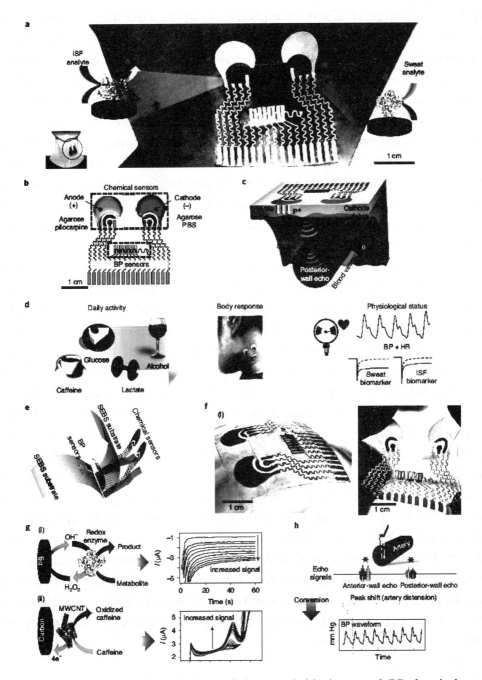

Fig. 10-1 | Design and mechanism of the stretchable integrated BP-chemical sensing patch. **a,** Illustrations of the placement of the sensor and the enzymatic chemical sensors for ISF and sweat. **b,** Illustration of the acoustic and electrochemical sensing components of the sensor along with hydrogels for sweat stimulation (left) and ISF extraction (right), respectively. **c,** Acoustic sensing and IP mechanism of the integrated sensor. The transducer applies ultrasound pulses that generate echoes from the anterior and posterior walls of the artery. Chemical sensing starts with the application of an IP current from a positive terminal (anode) to a negative terminal (cathode), which allows the electro-repulsive delivery of a sweat-stimulating molecule (P+, pilocarpine nitrate). After pilocarpine delivery, stimulated sweat-containing biomarkers (such as lactate, caffeine and alcohol) are collected and quantified on the left-hand side of the device. The IP current leads to osmotic flow of the biomarkers (such as glucose) from the ISF to the skin surface, allowing its collection and analysis on the right-hand side of the sensor. **d,** Schematics showing the different daily activities performed by an individual, labelled with their related biomarkers (alcohol, caffeine, lactate and glucose), followed by their effects on the physiological behaviour of an individual (body response). The inputs are transduced and outputted as BP, HR and electrochemical signals by the device, reflecting the physiological status of the body. **e,** The layer-by-layer layout of the integrated sensor. **f,** Photos of the sensor under bending (i) and stretching (ii). **g,** Mechanisms of detection for the electrochemical sensors. (i) Amperometric measurements using enzyme-based sensors. The Prussian-blue (PB) working electrode was modified with the redox enzymes lactate oxidase, glucose oxidase or alcohol oxidase, allowing the biocatalytic oxidation of lactate, glucose or alcohol molecules to pyruvate, gluconic acid or acetaldehyde (products), respectively, along with the production of hydrogen peroxide. The typical electrochemical reduction of the liberated hydrogen peroxide to hydroxyl ions (left) was performed in PBS pH 7.4 by applying a potential of -0.2 V. An increase in negative current is observed by an increase in the concentration of the chemical analyte (right). (ii) Caffeine non-enzymatic measurements. Caffeine was oxidized during the sensing process, which resulted in the production of uric-acid analogue molecules and electrons (left). A carbon electrode modified with multi-walled carbon nanotubes (MWCNT) allowed the pulse-voltammetric detection of caffeine following 30 s accumulation at -1.2 V and scanning between $+0.5$ V and $+1.5$ V; potential step, 0.004 V; pulse amplitude, 0.05 V; pulse width, 0.05 s; and scan rate, 0.02 V s-1. Following an increase in the concentration of caffeine, an increase in the oxidation signal is observed (right). **h,** Signal-generation mechanism of the ultrasound transducer (top). The pulsed ultrasound signal from the transducer is reflected from the anterior and posterior walls of the artery and collected by the transducer. Signal processing of the ultrasound signal (bottom). The time of flight of the reflected echo can be converted into BP via established transfer functions.

Outlook

Such acoustic and electrochemical sensing offers continuous monitoring of the physiological status of the user and its response to multiple everyday activities and stimuli. This multimodal wearable technology has thus been shown to be useful for correlating common daily activities—such as, exercise, drinking and eating—with changes in BP, HR and biomarker levels. These encouraging results support the possibility of developing hybrid wearable sensors with complex integration of chemical and physical sensors on a single conformal wearable patch for the simultaneous monitoring of multiple relevant parameters. Such integration of reliable and comprehensive epidermal sensors can only be realized with judicious selection of materials, optimized structural engineering and a high-throughput fabrication process in mind. Although the integrated device displays attractive features, there are still opportunities for the following improvements to the measurements of BP, HR and metabolites. (i) The integrated patch relies on the IP pilocarpine stimulation of sweat, which limits the operational use due to the depletion of pilocarpine. Long-term sweat-stimulating drugs (for example, carbachol) could be used to extend the operation period and perform multiple measurements using a single sweat-stimulation step. (ii) Testing of multiplexed patch designs to allow for comprehensive multi-analyte monitoring. (iii) Incorporation of a perspiration-rate sensing interface to normalize the ISF marker readings or use of sweat-suppressive drugs along with an internal standard (sodium) to address potential ISF dilution by passive sweating. (iv) Conducting extensive validations involving a large number of individuals with various health conditions, including patients with diabetes and cardiovascular disease. (v) Full miniaturization of the device through the development of electronics with integrated ultrasound and multi-potentiostatic capabilities, along with signal processing and wireless transmission functionalities. Previous examples have shown the successful miniaturization of wearable devices featuring multiplexed sensing modalities, wireless communications and displays. The future development of a stand-alone acoustic sensing interface circuit, coupled with artificial intelligence-aided signal processing, will fully transform the present device into a comprehensive skin-worn sensing system. By addressing these opportunities and adding more sensing parameters, we envision a fully integrated multiplexed wearable health-monitoring device that offers insights into the health and physiological status of individuals in the prevention and management of chronic diseases. This device represents a first step towards multimodal wearable sensors that fuse acoustic and electrochemical sensors for more comprehensive monitoring of human physiology and towards telehealth transformation. It thus paves the way into a family of skin-conformal tools capable of providing high-quality and high-density information regarding the status of human health and lays the foundation for next-generation wearable patches capable of hybrid chemical-electrophysiological-physical monitoring.

(This article is excerpted from "An epidermal patch for the simultaneous monitoring of haemodynamic and metabolic biomarkers" published in *Nature biomedical engineering*, PMID: 33589782)

Notes

1. telehealth: *n.* health care provided remotely to a patient in a separate location using two-way voice and visual communication (as by computer or cell phone); telemedicine 远程医疗

Words and Expressions

1. non-invasive: *adj.* relating to a technique that does not involve puncturing the skin or entering a body cavity 无创的

2. optimize: *v.* to improve the way that something is done or used so that it is as effective as possible 优化

3. resiliency: *n.* the ability of a substance to return to its original shape after it has been pressed or bent 弹性

4. crosstalk: *n.* unwanted signals in a communication channel (as in a telephone, radio, or computer) caused by transference of energy from another circuit (as by leakage or coupling) 串扰；串音

5. compensate: *v.* to give something good to balance or lessen the bad effect of damage 补偿

6. depletion: *n.* the state when an amount of something is greatly reduced or nearly all used up 消耗，用尽

7. intertwine: *v.* to be closely connected with（使）紧密相关

8. modality: *n.* the particular way in which something exists, is experienced or is done 形式；样式

9. integrate: *v.* to become closely linked or form part of a whole idea or system 整合

10. hybrid: *n.* a mixture of two or more distinct elements 混合物

11. fluctuation: *n.* a change in a price, amount, level etc.波动

12. conformal: *adj.* describing a mathematical transformation that leaves the angles between intersecting curves unchanged 保角的；保形的

13. judicious: *adj.* showing or having good sense 明智的

Medical Vocabulary

haemodynamic: 血液动力的

interstitial fluid: 间质液；组织液

glycolysis: 糖酵解

electrolyte: 电解液；电解质

septic: 脓毒性的

hypoglycemia: 低血糖症

hyperglycemia: 高血糖症

retinopathy: 视网膜病变

nephropathy: 肾病

piezoelectric lead zirconate titanate: 压电锆钛酸铅

solvent-soldering: 溶剂焊接

iontophoresis: 电离子透入疗法

styrene-ethylene-butylene-styrene block copolymer: 苯乙烯-乙烯-丁烯-苯乙烯嵌段共聚物

substrate: 基质

carotid artery: 颈动脉

enzymatic: 酶的

pilocarpine: 匹鲁卡品；毛果芸香碱（一种眼科缩瞳药）

redox: 氧化还原

oxidase: 氧化酶

pyruvate: 丙酮酸盐

acetaldehyde: 乙醛

hydrogen peroxide: 过氧化氢

potentiostatic: 恒电势的

Exercise

Critical Thinking

This article introduces the non-invasive skin-worn patch for simultaneously monitoring multiple relevant parameters. Please summarize the features and advantages of this hybrid device and discuss potential improvements with your partner.

Supplementary Reading

For more information on Smart Military Medical Technology, please go to the following websites:

1. https://www.telegraph.co.uk/education/stem-awards/defence-technology/augmented-reality-in-the-military/

2. https://www.forbes.com/sites/forbestechcouncil/2020/03/09/wearing-it-well-the-next-steps-for-wearable-medical-technology/?sh=334e0ea28d1a

3. https://www.electronicsforu.com/market-verticals/aerospace-defence/modern-sensors-defence-military-applications

参考译文

第一章　一切为了世界和平

课文 A　中国军队：联合国维和行动的关键力量

今年是中国人民抗日战争暨世界反法西斯战争胜利 75 周年，是联合国成立 75 周年，是中国军队参加联合国维和行动 30 周年。

30 年来，中国军队派出维和官兵的数量和类型全面发展，从最初的军事观察员，发展到工兵分队、医疗分队、运输分队、直升机分队、警卫分队、步兵营等成建制部队以及参谋军官、军事观察员、合同制军官等维和军事专业人员。中国维和官兵的足迹遍布柬埔寨、刚果（金）、利比里亚、苏丹、黎巴嫩、塞浦路斯、南苏丹、马里、中非等 20 多个国家和地区，在推进和平解决争端、维护地区安全稳定、促进驻在国经济社会发展等方面做出了重要贡献。

1. 监督停火

监督停火旨在确保冲突各方履行停火协议，是联合国维和行动的初始职能，也是中国军队承担的首项联合国维和任务。自 1990 年起，以军事观察员、参谋军官、合同制军官等为代表的中国维和军事专业人员队伍不断发展壮大。30 年来，中国军队累计向 25 个维和特派团及联合国总部派出维和军事专业人员 2064 人次。迄今，共有 13 名中国军人担任特派团司令、副司令，战区司令、副司令等重要职务。2020 年 8 月，有 84 名维和军事专业人员活跃在维和特派团和联合国总部，主要担负巡逻观察、监督停火、联络谈判、行动指挥、组织计划等任务。

军事观察员部署在冲突一线，为维和行动决策提供信息，经常受到武装冲突威胁。2006 年 7 月 25 日，黎以冲突期间，中国军事观察员杜照宇在炮火中坚守岗位履行职责，为和平事业献出了年轻的生命，被追记一等功，并被联合国授予哈马舍尔德勋章。

2. 稳定局势

迅速稳定局势是推进和平进程的前提条件，是联合国维和特派团的主要任务，也是近年来中国维和部队职能拓展的重要方向。部分维和任务区安全形势严峻，各类冲突不断，恐怖袭击、暴力骚乱频发。在各类维和分队中，步兵营主要执行武装巡逻、隔离冲突、止暴平暴、警戒搜查等任务，是维和行动的主力军、安全局势的"稳定器"。

2015 年 1 月，中国军队向联合国南苏丹特派团（联南苏团）派遣 1 支 700 人规模的步兵营，这是中国军队首次成建制派遣步兵营赴海外执行维和任务。5 年来，中国军队先后向南苏丹派遣 6 批维和步兵营。迎着朝霞出发、披着星光归营，在枪声中入睡、在炮声中惊醒，这是维和步兵营官兵工作生活的真实写照。截至 2020 年 8 月，维和步兵营累计完成长途巡逻 51 次、短途巡逻 93 次，武装护卫任务 314 次，武器禁区巡逻 3 万余小时，为稳定当地局势发挥了重要作用。2018 年 8 月，南苏丹首都朱巴发生大规模械斗流血事件。中国维和步兵营奉命出击，果断处置，迅速平息事态。

3. 保护平民

保护平民是联合国维和行动的重要内容，也是中国维和官兵义不容辞的责任、义无反顾的抉择。近代以来，中国人民饱受战乱之苦，中国官兵深知和平之宝贵、生命之无价。在战火频仍的维和任务区，中国维和官兵用汗水和青春浇灌美丽的和平之花，用热血和生命撑起一片片和平的蓝天。

2016 年 7 月，南苏丹首都朱巴爆发武装冲突，政府军和反政府武装持续激战，双方投入坦克、大口径火炮、武装直升机等重型武器，身处交火地域的大量平民生命安全受到严重威胁。中国维和步兵营及友邻部队共同承担辖区内朱巴城区及城郊百余村庄平民的安全保护任务。面对枪林弹雨，中国维和官兵用血肉之躯构筑"生命防线"，阻止武装分子接近平民保护区，守护了 9000 多名平民的生命安全。执行任务期间，李磊、杨树朋两名战士壮烈牺牲，用生命履行使命，以英勇无畏践行了保护生命、捍卫和平的铮铮誓言，被追记一等功，并被联合国授予哈马舍尔德勋章。

4. 安全护卫

安全护卫是确保联合国特派团设施和人员安全的重要任务。中国军队作为联合国维和行动的重要参与者，积极派出维和安全部队，为联合国维和行动提供有力的安全保障。

2013 年 12 月，中国军队向联合国马里多层面综合稳定特派团（联马团）派遣 1 支170 人的警卫分队，承担联马团东战区司令部安全警戒、要员护卫等任务，这是中国军队首次派遣安全部队参与维和行动。马里是联合国最危险的维和任务区之一，自杀式袭击、路边炸弹等恐袭事件屡屡发生。7 年来，中国军队先后向马里维和任务区派遣 8 批警卫分队、官兵 1440 人次，在危机四伏的撒哈拉沙漠南缘，警卫分队官兵出色完成任务，累计执行武装巡逻及警戒护卫等行动 3900 余次，被联马团东战区誉为"战区王牌"。2016年 5 月 31 日，中国维和士兵申亮亮为阻止载有炸药的恐怖分子车辆冲入联合国维和营地壮烈牺牲，被追记一等功，并被联合国授予哈马舍尔德勋章。中华人民共和国成立 70周年之际，申亮亮烈士被授予"人民英雄"国家荣誉称号。

2017 年 3 月 12 日，南苏丹边境城镇耶伊爆发激烈冲突，7 名联合国民事人员被困在交火区域中心，生命安全面临严重威胁。中国赴南苏丹维和步兵营火速派出 12 名官兵前往救援。行进途中险情不断，救援官兵临危不惧，与武装分子斗智斗勇，3 次突破拦截，成功将全部被困民事人员安全转移。此次救援行动及时高效，被联南苏团作为解救行动成功范例加以推广。

5. 支援保障

工程、运输、医疗、直升机等后勤保障分队在联合国维和行动中扮演着不可或缺的重要角色，是当前中国军队向海外派遣维和部队的主体。在各维和任务区，中国后勤保障分队官兵以过硬的素质、精湛的技能和敬业的精神，创造了"中国质量""中国速度""中国标准"等一块块闪亮的中国品牌。

2020 年 1 月，联马团北战区泰萨利特维和营地遭到恐怖袭击，造成 20 多人受伤。部署在东战区的中国医疗分队紧急前出，将 7 名乍得维和部队伤员接回至中国医疗分队。经过全力抢救，所有伤员转危为安。2020 年 5 月，中国维和工兵分队克服新冠肺炎疫情防控压力大、安全形势严峻等不利因素，高标准、高质量完成南苏丹西部索普桥修建，打通瓦乌至拉加线路，赢得当地政府和人民的高度评价和赞誉。

30 年来，中国军队先后向柬埔寨、刚果（金）、利比里亚、苏丹、黎巴嫩、苏丹达尔富尔、南苏丹、马里 8 个维和任务区派遣 111 支工兵分队 25768 人次，累计新建和修复道路 1.7 万多千米、桥梁 300 多座，排除地雷及未爆炸物 1.4 万余枚，完成大量平整场地、维修机场、搭建板房、构筑防御工事等工程保障任务；先后向利比里亚、苏丹 2 个任务区派遣 27 支运输分队、5164 人次，累计运送物资器材 120 万余吨，运输总里程 1300 万余千米；先后向刚果（金）、利比里亚、苏丹、黎巴嫩、南苏丹、马里 6 个任务区派遣 85 支医疗分队、4259 人次，累计接诊救治病人、抢救伤员 24.6 万余人次；向苏丹达尔富尔派遣 3 支直升机分队、420 人次，累计飞行 1602 架次、1951 小时，运送人员 10410 人次、物资 480 余吨。

6. 播撒希望

过上幸福美好生活，是各国人民的共同期盼。远赴海外的中国维和官兵用实际行动，为遭受战火摧残的人民带去了和平、点亮了希望。

积极协助开展人道主义救援。30 年来，中国维和部队与国际人道主义机构携手，积极参与难民安置、救济粮发放、难民营修建和抢险救灾等行动，开展了大量卓有成效的工作。2020 年 4 月，刚果（金）东部乌维拉地区暴发罕见洪灾，人民生命财产安全面临严重威胁，中国工兵分队临危受命，紧急加固堤坝，修复被毁桥梁，打通生命通道，有力保护当地人民安全。

广泛参与战后重建。战乱国家或地区签署和平协议后，帮助其恢复社会秩序、改善民生，是防止冲突再起、实现持久和平与稳定的治本之策。中国维和部队积极参与驻地战后重建进程，承担重要基础设施援建、协助监督选举、医护人员培训及环境保护等任务，得到驻在国政府和人民的积极评价。苏丹达尔富尔地区地处沙漠边缘、地质结构复杂，是世界上极度贫水的地区之一，2007 年至 2013 年期间，中国工兵分队给水官兵克服重重困难，先后在当地打井 14 口，有效缓解当地人民的饮水难题。

传递温暖和爱心。中国维和官兵不仅是和平的守护人，也是友谊的传播者。中国赴刚果（金）医疗分队与驻地布卡武市"国际儿童村"结成对子，用真情传递爱心和温暖，中国女官兵被孩子们亲切称作"中国妈妈"，这一爱心接力棒已经接续了 17 年，在当地传为佳话。中国赴南苏丹维和部队向当地人民传授农业技术、赠送农具菜种，并应邀到当地中学开设中国文化和汉语课程，深受学生们欢迎。

30 年来，中国军队先后参加 25 项联合国维和行动，累计派出维和官兵 4 万余人次，16 名中国官兵为了和平事业献出了宝贵生命。2020 年 8 月，2521 名中国官兵正在 8 个维和特派团和联合国总部执行任务。中国女性维和官兵在维和行动中发挥了越来越重要的作用，先后有 1000 余名女性官兵参与医疗保障、联络协调、扫雷排爆、巡逻观察、促进性别平等、妇女儿童保护等工作，展示了中国女性的巾帼风采。中国维和部队的出色表现，受到联合国高度认可，赢得国际社会广泛赞赏，为国家和军队赢得了荣誉。

第二章 联合国卫勤保障

课文 A 维和行动中的卫勤保障

联合国维和行动中的卫勤保障任务表述是：通过对任务区内医疗保健进行规划、协调、实施、监测和专业监管，维护联合国维和行动人员的健康和安全。

1. 结构组织

维和部队内部指挥体系清晰明了，任务区最高医务官，即部队医务官（FMedO）直接隶属于维和部队指挥官（FC）或指定的特派团团长。部队医务官全权代表维和部队指挥官处理一切与医疗相关的事务，并统管任务区内所有联合国战地医疗所，其提供的医疗服务覆盖整个部队。他还负责对各派遣国分遣队下属的建制医疗分队进行业务上的监管，后者的指挥权仍归属各国分遣部队指挥官。同理，部队医务官在政策和具体操作事宜上分别受联合国总部医疗服务司与卫勤保障股的监管。上述各机构紧密协作，确保为任务区提供有效的卫勤保障。联合国卫勤保障组织如图 2-1 所示。

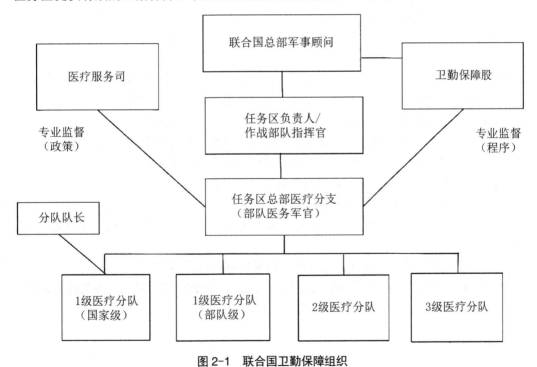

图 2-1 联合国卫勤保障组织

2. 联合国卫勤保障分级

联合国维和任务卫勤保障具有标准化的分级体系，以确保向维和人员提供最高水平的医疗保障，尤其是考虑到医疗分队和医护人员来自不同国家，其医疗护理标准各不相同，因此这种标准化的分级体系非常必要。联合国卫勤保障分级如下：

2.1 基础级卫勤保障

基础级卫勤保障是指在最小的次分队级别实施的基本急救和预防保健。该级别没有医生，医疗救治由维和人员或受过训练的护理员或护士承担，借助基本的医疗设备和器材完成。表2-1列出了基础级卫勤保障在培训和设备保障方面的要求。

表2-1　基础级卫勤保障

救治范围	治疗能力	设备要求	备注
-非医务人员或护理员实施的急救 -核心技能： 1. 心肺复苏 2. 出血控制 3. 骨折固定 4. 伤口包扎（包括烧伤） 5. 伤员运输和后送 6. 通信和报告		-急救包 -个人野战包扎敷料 -口袋型呼吸面罩（可选）	-由各派遣国负责对所派维和人员进行培训，确保其掌握必需的医护技能 -应按照卫勤保障股（MSU）制定的相关标准组织维和人员进行医护技能培训

2.2 一级卫勤保障

一级卫勤保障是有医生在场的第一个级别的卫勤保障，包括一线初级医疗护理、急救复苏、伤员稳定及伤员后送（至维和任务区内上一级卫勤保障单位）。

一级医疗单位具体任务如下：

a）为700人（及以下）规模的维和部队提供初级医疗保健，每天诊治至少20名非卧床病员。

b）为尚未进行体检的维和人员进行入职体检，必要时可安排进行其他相关检查。

c）进行局麻条件下的简单外科处理，例如清创缝合、脓肿切开。

d）进行急救复苏，例如保持气道和呼吸通畅、止血、抗休克。

e）对伤员进行验伤分诊，稳定其生命体征，并将其后送至上一级医疗单位。

f）住院收治最多5名伤员，每人住院观察、治疗时间最多2天。

g）实施免疫接种和任务区要求的其他疾病预防措施。

h）进行基本的战地诊断和化验检测。

i）随时有能力拆分成两个独立的先遣医疗队（FTMs），可同时在两处地点提供医疗保障。

j）监督其保障范围内部队和人员预防保健措施的执行情况。

一级医疗分队需配备可供60天使用的充足的医疗物资和消耗品。有关救治范围、人员、设备和基础设施方面的具体信息如表2-2。

表 2-2　一级卫勤保障

救治范围	治疗能力	人员要求	设备要求	基础设施
1. 常见疾病治疗 2. 高级生命支持 　-维持气道开放 　-人工通气 　-出血控制 　-休克和脱水的救治 3. 外伤处置 　-骨折固定 　-创伤和烧伤处理 　-感染控制 　-镇痛	-每天治疗 20 名门诊患者 -收治 5 名留观最多 2 天的患者 -最多 60 天的医用物资和消耗品储备	2 名军医官 6 名护理员/护士 3 名保障人员 注：有能力拆分为 2 个先遣医疗组，每组含 1 名医生、2-3 名护理人员	-用于复苏和生命维持的设备、液体和药物 -战地药房 -用于门诊和病房的整套设备 -小型外科手术所需的外科器材 -夹板、绷带和担架 -医生/护理人员装备便携式卫生包/囊 -基础野外检验箱 -消毒设备和冰箱 -1-2 辆救护车	-帐篷或方舱 -房屋建筑（如有） -一般性基础保障和办公设施

2.3　二级卫勤保障

二级卫勤保障是更高一级的医疗保障，也是具备专业外科治疗力量和设施的第一级医疗保障。二级医疗机构的任务是提供第二线医疗保健、急救复苏和稳定、以挽救肢体和生命为目的的外科干预手术、基本口腔保健及伤员后送（至上一级医疗单位）。

二级医疗单位的任务包括：

a）为 1000 人（及以下）规模的维和部队提供初级医疗保健，每天诊治最多 40 名非卧床病员。

b）按照要求组织实施维和人员入职体检以及常规例行体检，必要时可安排进行其他相关检查。

c）实施以挽救肢体和生命为目的的手术，如剖腹检查、阑尾切除、胸腔穿刺、创口开放和清创、骨折固定和截除，要求具备每天实施 3-4 台全麻大型手术的能力。

d）实施急救复苏，如维持气道开放、维持呼吸及血液循环、高级生命支持、出血控制和其他挽救肢体和生命的急救措施。

e）对伤员进行验伤分诊，稳定其生命体征，并将其后送至上一级医疗单位。

f）住院收治最多 20 名伤员，每人住院治疗、护理时间最多 7 天，同时可为 1-2 名病人提供重症监护护理。

g）实施基础 X 线检查，上限为每天 10 例。

h）实施牙科治疗，上限为每天 10 例，包括止痛、拔牙、补牙和感染控制。

i）实施免疫接种，并根据任务区要求，实施其他疾病预防措施。

j）进行化验室检验检测，上限为每天 20 例，包括血常规、血生化和尿常规。

k）组建、部署至少 2 个先遣医疗组（每组包括 1 名军医和 2 名护理人员），赴二级救助点提供医疗护理和保健，或在地面及空中后送行动中提供卫勤保障。

l）维持足够 60 天使用的医用物资和消耗品储备，并有能力在必要时帮助任务区内一级医疗单位，为其提供再补给。

二级医疗分队的救治范围、治疗能力，以及所需人员和装备的具体要求如表 2-3 所示。

表2-3 二级卫勤保障

救治范围	治疗能力	人员要求	设备要求	基础设施
1. 常见病治疗 2. 分级诊疗 3. 高级生命支持和重症监护 4. 麻醉情况下保全生命和肢体的外科手术 5. 药房 6. 基础牙科治疗 7. 基础检验检测设施 -血型和交叉配血 -血液学 -革兰氏染色 -血涂片 -尿常规 8. 基础放射学诊断 9. 卫生管理和预防保健 10. 后送伤员至第三或第四级医疗单位	-每天门诊接诊能力上限为40人 -每天3—4台大型手术 -收治10—20名住院病人，每人住院治疗时间不超过7天 -每天5—10例牙科治疗 -每天10例X线检查和20例实验室检验检测 -60天的医用物资和消耗品储备	2名外科医生（普外和矫形外科） 1名麻醉师 1名内科医师 1名全科医生 1名牙科医生 1名卫生检验专员 1名药师 1名护士长 2名ICU护士 1名康复治疗师 10名护士/护理员 1名放射科技师 1名化验员 1名牙科医助 2名司机 8名保障人员 总计：35人	-门诊和病房设备 -急救室设备 -标准手术室器材设备 -重症监护设备 -野外检验检测和放射设备 -牙科治疗椅和其他设备 -医院需要的其他保障设备如：高压灭菌器、冰箱、救护车2台	1. 医院 -接待/行政室 -急救室 -门诊诊室 -病房1—2间 -带1—2个床位的ICU病房 -手术室 -药房 -X线室 -化验室 -牙科区 -消毒区 2. 保障勤务 -厨房 -洗衣房 -储藏设备 -维修设施 -通信设施 -发电机 -办公室 -公共卫生和垃圾处理设备 -宿舍和食堂

2.4 三级卫勤保障

三级卫勤保障是联合医疗队负责提供的最高一级卫勤保障。它集一级、二级医疗单位的救治范围于一身，并增加了专科住院治疗、手术以及全面的诊疗服务。需要注意的是，联合国极少部署三级医疗分队，通常该级别的保障通过任务区内或邻近国家现有的地方或军队医院来实现。

三级医疗分队的任务如下：

a）为5000人（及以下）规模的维和部队提供初级医疗保健，每天诊治至少60名非卧床病员。

b）提供专科医疗咨询服务，特别是在内科、传染病、热带医学、皮肤病、心理疾病和妇科等领域。

c）实施全麻条件下大型普外或矫形外科手术，上限为每天10例，如有外科专科医生主刀更佳，如神经外科、心胸外科、创伤外科、泌尿外科、烧伤科等。

d）实施急救复苏，如维持气道开放、维持呼吸及血液循环、高级生命支持。

e）稳定伤员生命体征，使其在长距离空中后送过程中保持病情稳定，能够顺利到达可能位于另一个国家的四级医疗机构。

f）住院收治最多50名伤员，每人住院治疗、护理时间最多30天，同时可为最多4名病人提供重症监护护理。

g）实施基础基本放射（X线）检查，上限为每天20例，如能提供超声或CT扫描则更佳。

h）实施牙科治疗，每天10－20例，包括止痛、拔牙、补牙和感染控制，以及局部口腔手术。

i）实施免疫接种，并根据任务区要求，实施其他疾病预防措施。

j）进行化验室检验检测，上限为每天40例。

k）组建、部署至少2个先遣医疗组（每组包括1名军医和2名护理人员），赴二级救助点提供医疗护理和保健，或在地面及空中后送（包括螺旋桨和固定翼飞机实施的空中后送）行动中提供卫勤保障。

l）维持足够60天使用的医用物资和消耗品储备，并有能力在必要时帮助任务区内一级、二级医疗单位，为其提供有限的再补给。

三级医疗分队的救治范围、治疗能力，以及所需人员、装备、基础设施等细节情况如表2-4所示。

表2-4　三级卫勤保障

救治范围	治疗能力	人员要求	装备要求	基础设施
涵盖二级医疗保障分队所有救治范围，此外还包括： 1. 专科咨询服务 2. 多学科外科治疗 3. 术后和重症监护 4. 全套实验室检验检测 5. 放射学诊断（配备超声和CT扫描设备更佳） 6. 药房 7. 口腔外科和口腔X线	-每天门诊接诊能力上限为60人 -每天不超过10台大手术 -最多收治50名住院病人，每人住院治疗时间不超过30天 -每天10－20例牙科治疗 -每天20例X线检查和40例实验室检验检测 -60天的医用物资和消耗品储备	16名医生，包括： -普外科医生 -矫形外科医生 -麻醉师 -内科医生 -全科医生 -皮肤科医生 -精神科医生 -其他专科医生 1名口腔外科医生 1名牙医 2名牙科医助 1名卫生检验专员 1名药师 1名药师助理 50名护理人员，包括： -护士长 -ICU护士 -康复治疗师 -护士 -护理员 2名放射科技师 2名化验员 14名保障人员 总计：91人	同二级医疗单位所需设备，此外还包括： -普外科和整形外科手术室器材设备 -重症和高依赖性监护设备 -实验室和放射科设备 -牙科治疗椅和牙科X线设备 -救护车 -普通运输设备	1. 医院 -接待/行政室 -急救室 -门诊室4间 -病房2－4间 -带4张床位的ICU病房 -手术室2间 -药房 -X线室 -化验室 -口腔外科（2张治疗椅） -口腔X线室 -消毒室 2. 保障勤务 -厨房 -洗衣房 -储藏设备 -维修设施 -通信设施 -发电机 -燃料储存室 -水质净化 -公共卫生和垃圾处理设备 -宿舍和食堂

2.5 四级卫勤保障

四级卫勤保障机构负责提供终极医疗护理和专科治疗，这些保障内容在任务区内目前没有或无可行条件给予提供，包括专科手术和治疗、重建、修复和康复。此类治疗专业性要求和费用都比较高，并且有可能需要较长的治疗周期，因此对于联合国来说，在任务区内部署此类机构既不实用又不经济。此类医疗服务通常借助在驻国、邻国或派遣国国内的医疗单位来实现。联合国可安排将伤病员后送到此类机构。同时，出于成本、补偿和抚恤金等方面的考虑，联合国也将继续跟踪病人的病情进展。

当以下情况出现时，说明联合国医务人员可动用四级医疗保障服务：

a）任务区距本土太远，且伤病员病情危急，急需专科治疗。

b）患者仅需短期专科治疗，且部队要求该患者 30 天内归队。

c）派遣国没有能力提供对症的终极治疗（不包括维和人员被派遣到任务区前已确诊或已经正在接受治疗的慢性病）。

d）联合国已收到某国提出提供终极治疗的申请，包括已与相关国家签署合同或协助通知书，且已安排划拨适当金额的经费。

2.6 先遣医疗队

先遣医疗队是规模小而机动性极高的医疗单元，大约由 3 人组成，其人员构成和装备主要针对短期野外卫勤保障，一般是在有需要时临时由任务区内已有医疗单位抽组形成（包括人员、设备和补给品），但也可以是应派遣国要求成立并部署的一个独立单位，有单独的任务。先遣医疗队所有的勤务保障需求都依靠它们保障的单位来满足。

先遣医疗队的任务包括：

a）在医疗站保障大约 100-150 人的独立军事特遣队，为其提供初级医疗护理和应急医疗服务。

b）在无联合国医疗设施可供直接使用的地区为短期野战行动提供一线卫勤保障。

c）在地面和/或空中伤员（尤其是伤情严重或不稳定的伤员）后送期间、后送距离较长或很有可能出现延迟的情况下，为伤员提供持续的医疗护理。必要时还包括护送伤病员离开任务区，将其后送至附近国家或医疗遣返至派出国。

d）为搜救任务提供医疗队。

为保证在上述行动任务中有效运行，先遣医疗队（无论其规模大小如何）必须配备精良，包括配备生命支持相关的医疗设备。所有设备和用品都需要轻便便携，适合在救护车和直升机等密闭空间使用。

第三章　联合国维和行动中的医疗救治

课文 A　伤员救治与后送

1. 分诊

分诊是根据临床评估对患者或伤员进行分类，目的是确定治疗和后送的优先顺序。这有助于有效利用有限的医疗资源，并在多人伤亡的情况下尽可能确保更多的人活下来。

分诊通常由最有经验的医生或护理人员进行。这是一个持续的过程，因为伤员的状况可能会恶化，特别是在后送期间。分诊应在到达医疗机构后进行，并在后送进一步治疗之前再次进行。

1.1 分类

国际和国家卫生保健组织采用了不同的分诊分类方法。有些是根据患者或伤员后送或治疗的紧急程度对其进行分类，同时也要考虑到他/她可能的预后情况。一些分类系统是基于创伤评分，而其他一些系统主要取决于临床判断。医疗单位必须熟悉任务区内其他单位的分诊分类标准和标签。

1.2 分诊类别

联合国建议根据医疗状况的严重程度和治疗的紧迫性采用四类分诊命名法。

a）第一优先级（红色：立即）：此类别对治疗或后送具有最高优先级，因为需要紧急后送干预以确保伤员或患者的生存。包括气道阻塞、呼吸急症、休克和严重创伤。如果得不到适当的医疗救治，此类病例很可能会在 2 小时或更短的时间内死亡。

b）第二优先级（黄色：紧急）：这包括需要早期治疗的疾病，特别是需要手术的，建议在受伤后 6 小时内转移到外科机构。包括内脏损伤、没有窒息威胁的闭合性胸部损伤、重大肢体损伤和骨折、闭合性头部损伤、眼部外伤和中度烧伤。

c）第三优先级（绿色：延迟或后送）：此级别的治疗不太紧急，如果有其他伤亡人员需要有限的治疗或后送资源，则可以推迟此级别的治疗。包括简单的闭合性骨折、软组织损伤、闭合性胸部损伤和上颌面部损伤。

d）第四优先级（黑色：濒临死亡或死亡）：此级别是指受伤或疾病非常严重，生存机会很小或在抵达时已死亡。如果存在对有限医疗资源的竞争，尽管病情严重，其后送或治疗优先级较低。例如脑干死亡和绝症。

2. 治疗和收容政策

2.1 医疗机构提供的治疗取决于其卫勤保障级别。级别较低的，其重点在于伤员的复苏及稳定以利于向后一级后送。对于重伤的情况，该级别很少提供确定性救治，主要是尽量避免耽误继续后送。

2.2 任务区内医疗资源的组织由各级救治和后送能力决定。如果预计后送有困难或延迟，这些级别必须相应地具有更大的处理能力。任务中的收容政策（也称为后送政策）用于平衡每级的救治能力与可提供的后送资源。这通过规定伤病员可以在每级留治的最长时间来决定，之后如果他不能返回工作岗位，他将被后送。该政策由以下因素决定：

a）因后送资源不可用、行动受限、天气或地形而导致的后送受阻。

b）对医疗资源的需求，例如预计会有大量病员，留治时间可能会缩短。

c）医疗物资的可用性，例如在任务开始或结束时，设备相对较少，留治时间相对较短。

3. 医疗后送和遣返

3.1 维和行动部的计划参谋和任务区内的行政、卫生参谋负责计划和建立有效的医疗后送体系。在任务行政管理部门的支持和医疗服务司的指导下，部队医务官协调所有的维和区内的后送行动。后送计划的细节包含在每个任务标准行动程序（SOP）内。有三类疾病/伤员转移方式：

a）伤员后送：将伤员从受伤地点向最近的医疗机构后送，理想的时机为受伤后 1 小时内。

b）医疗后送：两级医疗分队之间的伤员后送，可以是任务区内或者是任务区外的，伤员可按照收容政策规定的时间表归队或被遣返。

c）医疗遣返：因医疗原因，伤病员返回其祖国，其后他不再回到任务区。

3.2 制定计划

a）任务收容政策。如上所述，任务收容政策必须在任务开始时就制定，它确定伤病员在每级医疗分队留置的最长时间（天），之后决定每级医疗分队的治疗能力和范围以及所需要的后送能力。

b）后送指征。伤病员的临床表现是决定各级之间后送的时间和方式的关键指标。

c）救治机构的后送时机。必须及时后送，允许患者尽可能早地获得所需的生命或肢体抢救措施，建议伤员到二级或三级医疗分队的时间不得超过受伤后 4 小时。

d）空运后送。虽然可能不总使用空运，最理想的还是由直升机进行医疗后送，由配有基本维持生命装备和供给的先遣医疗组实施。如果在任务区内没有二级和/或三级医疗分队，就必须尽快利用直升机或飞机后送到这些机构。

3.3 医疗后送

如果当地的救治机构不能提供必需的治疗，就要考虑医疗后送。其政策和程序如下：

a）国际征募官员、军事和文职人员由联合国支付后送费用，目的是确保获得在任务区内得不到但又是必需的医疗护理；当地征募的官员及其配偶和没有独立生活的子女，在紧急状况下即医疗风险很高或生命受到威胁时也可后送。

b）紧急情况下，在与部队医务官和行政主任军官商议后，任务首长或部队指挥官可以直接授权医疗后送，在任务区内实施时，不必事先征求联合国总部的同意。

c）可经陆路或空运进行后送，应当送往责任区内最近的合适的医疗机构，也应考虑其疾病和外伤的情况、所需治疗的类型和所使用语言的情况，所使用的运输工具最好清楚地标有红十字/红新月标志。

d）后送前和飞行时对患者的治疗必须要做充分的记录，并随病人至后一级救治机构，如果需要，可批准医生或护士陪伴。

e）由于分娩、精神疾病而需要延长康复时间的，要鼓励后送到其家乡休假或遣返回国。

f）如果伤员反对到推荐的后送地点，更喜欢到他/她的家乡休假，将首选批准后送到其家乡。

g）如果某国更倾向于后送自己的人员，但与负责的医官或部队医务官的意见相左时，便由该国负责并由其支付费用。

h）非紧急情况下，在医疗后送之前要寻求联合国总部的批准；紧急情况下，不需要批准，但其后要立即通知联合国总部。后送情况要上报后勤司和联合国医疗司司长。

i）在主治医生签署康复文件后，签署件的副本应交给医疗服务司司长，司长将确定其是否能归队。严重疾病和外伤的情况下，由联合国付费的患者在得到医疗司司长批准之前，可以不归队。但非紧急时不适用此条。

j）军事人员的医疗后送程序必须详尽地列入任务标准作业程序。联合国官员医疗后送的条款应在联合国野外行政手册中列出，也可在修订的 ST/AI 有关医疗后送中找到更多的细节。

3.4 医疗遣返

医疗遣返是将伤员后送至他/她的祖国或原先工作的地方，有关遣返的政策和程序如下：

a）医疗原因的遣返通常适用于根据已有收容政策（后送政策）不适合返回其工作岗位的，或所在任务区内无法提供其所需诊疗的所有人员。收容期限通常为 30 天。

b）医疗遣返由部队医务官负责，相应国家的分遣队首长和行政主任军官进行配合。被遣返后人员的进一步治疗将由本国负责。

c）到达任务区的军事人员，如不能胜任职责将马上被遣返，费用由其国负担。如果遣返原因是被诊断为慢性病，或任命时正在接受治疗的，费用必须由派遣国承担。

d）怀孕妇女将在孕期满 5 个月被遣返。

e）所有有艾滋病临床症状和体征的人员必须被遣返。

f）遣返首先要获得医疗服务司司长的批准。不论费用由联合国、该国政府或个人负担，部队医务官或负责医生必须提交一个书面建议。一旦批准，行政主任军官用最经济的办法通过任务或分队组织遣返。

g）如果可能，正常轮转或定期的勤务航班应当用于遣返，旅行费和机场费由联合国支付，行李费用完全由个人支付。如需护送，仅限于航空公司同意免费时，并要服从现行制度和规定。

h）如果需要紧急医疗遣返，可与军用或民用飞机签约。自 1989 年起，联合国与瑞士政府就有关维和行动的空中救护运送签署了一个长期的协议，由瑞士空中救援队 REGA 提供服务，并规定后送期间由 REGA 提供卫生人员与装备。

4. 大批伤亡和灾难管理

本节仅讨论有关联合国人员的情况，而为当地居民提供的人道主义援助将另行考虑。任务区内的所有医疗分队必须为大批伤亡和灾难做好准备。在新任务开始时，必须制定应急事件处理计划并分配好资源，同时与任务的执行和安全计划协调一致。由现场小分队到分遣队总部、地区总部直至任务区总部，每一级都要有计划。

4.1 定义

大批伤亡和灾难是突发情况，需处理大量伤员，将会导致医疗资源不足，因此患病和死亡的可能性将上升。可能是由自然或人为造成，并可伴随大量的物资、基础设施和环境的损坏。

4.2 卫勤保障

a）紧急情况下，医疗分队将动用其所有的可用资源提供紧急保障，包括在事故发生现场开设急救站和常规治疗中心，以及保障搜救行动。

b）伤员分类对于建立治疗和后送优先权十分重要，后送可经由地面和空运到联合国、当地和非政府组织的医疗机构，集中协调与管理成员向这些医疗机构的后送也十分必要。

c）现场提供的治疗，将仅限于基础生命支持和伤员复苏，基本目标是稳定伤员伤情，并将其后送到有适当人员和设备的医疗机构。

d）有关伤员情况、伤情和治疗的简要资料应该伴随所有的伤员，如果可能，应该随带分类标签。

e）死者的处理也应有计划，包括（如果可能）当场验明身份。与当地政府密切协作是必要的，以确保处理、运送遗体以及最后验明和埋葬工作顺利。

4.3 计划指南

a）明确危险因素和潜在威胁，包括当地各派可能的敌对行动。

b）准备任务区可提供的医疗物资清单，包括后送工具和当地基础设施。

c）应急计划，包括医疗分队分组，界定责任区和个人任务，确定可能的伤员收容区域和后送路线。

d）建立行动中心，以集中调配医疗资源和协调后送。

e）通信计划，包括配备无线电设备，并与其他联合国机构、当局政府和非政府组织协调。

f）后勤保障，包括医疗物资供给。

g）特殊医疗要求，包括医疗情况汇报和对受害者、抢救人员和卫生人员的应急处理。

第四章 战伤救治

课文 A 战场外科护理的"十大"研发重点

美国军队目前实现了史上最高的伤亡存活率。然而，在战斗创伤方面，仍有多个领域对提供高质量且高效的创伤护理提出了挑战。

现代美国战场护理的组织和职责范围大致可分为三类：（1）伤点和院前护理；（2）运送至医疗机构期间的护理（途中护理）；（3）高级外科护理。尽管该系统的总体目标是提供从受伤到医疗后送出作战区的无缝护理，但是每个领域有其独特的能力、挑战和需求以提供最佳护理。解决这些领域知识缺乏或能力次优的问题一直是政府资助多个研发项目的核心重点，例如战伤救治研究项目（CCCRP）。为了确定适宜的研究目标并为其提供研究项目资金，以解决现有的"研究缺口"，必须使用一个可靠的体系来识别、表征这些缺口，并对其按优先级排序。

在最近的战斗经历中，可以说最重要的组织发展是建立了联合创伤系统（JTS），该系统执行广泛的过程质量改进计划，运营国防部创伤登记系统（DODTR），并支持战斗伤亡护理研究项目（CCCRP），帮助其确定关键研发重点。作为这些活动的重要参与部分，联合创伤系统（JTS）成立了三个委员会，其关注重点和责任领域与上述三个阶段的护理（院前护理、途中护理和高级外科护理）相对应。其中最早也可以说最为成功的是战术战伤救治委员会（CoTCCC）。该委员会的工作带来了战场创伤护理质量与标准化的重大改进，人们广泛认可该委员会是过去 15 年作战行动中病死率历史最低的一个关键因素。战术战伤救治委员会（CoTCCC）另一个里程碑式的工作成果是确定并公布了需要重点研发的缺口清单。自发布以来，这份"十大"名单一直是地方和军界研究人员和研究管理人员的宝贵资源。然而，这项成果主要集中在创伤当场和院前阶段的干预护理缺口上，没有解决随后护理阶段的不同问题或具体挑战。基于战术战伤救治委员会（CoTCCC）取得的重大成就，联合创伤系统（JTS）又成立了两个委员会：途中救护委员会（CoERCC），重点关注医疗运输和撤离阶段的护理；外科战伤救治委员会（CoSCCC），重点关注具有手术能力的医疗设施（MTF）所提供的护理（任务 2 或任务 3 护理）。

外科战伤救治委员会（CoSCCC）制定了一份关键"重点领域"清单。前五个重点领域是人员/人员配置、复苏与出血管理、疼痛/镇静/焦虑管理、手术干预以及初步评估。"十大"具体研究主题已经确定（由于第 10 位存在相同得分，实际共有 11 个主题），表 4-1 中列出了这些主题及其对应的重点领域。"十大"研究重点全部来自三个重点领域，其中四个研究重点属于人员/人员配置领域，四个研究重点属于复苏/出血管理领域，三个研究重点属于手术干预领域。

这是对战斗创伤护理研究重点的第一次客观排序。这些数据将有助于指导国防部的研究计划，优先资助军事和民用研究人员的新领域。

表 4-1　高级外科护理的"十大"研究重点

研究重点	重点领域	得分（均值）
1. 评估小型"简朴外科团队"和标准规模的高级外科团队的实际能力、潜在益处与危害	人员/人员配置	8.46
2. 优化血液制品及输血储存	复苏和初步出血管理	8.22
3. 针对各种任务/场景的最佳人员数量、组合与培训	人员/人员配置	8.17
4. 不可压迫性躯干出血的非手术干预治疗	复苏和初步出血管理	8.13
5. 失血性腹腔出血的损伤控制干预	手术干预	7.92
6. 手术室团队技能构成对手术效果的影响	手术干预	7.77
7. 基于单位规模结构的结果分析与比较	人员/人员配置	7.77
8. 主要血管损伤的损伤控制干预	手术干预	7.75
9. 手术病例负荷与构成分析，确定人员需求的必要技能	人员/人员配置	7.73
10A. 复苏性主动脉球囊阻断术——改进使用途径/方法、指导设备放置、监测有效性	复苏和初步出血管理	7.72
10B. 止血复苏的凝血因子浓缩制品与替代品	复苏和初步出血管理	7.72

人员与人员配置（数量、结构、能力）

令人惊讶的是，最优先的研究重点和重点领域都与非临床主题相关，即人员配备与高级外科能力。事实上，十大研究重点中有四项与人员和人员配置有关，我们认为，这体现出在近期变化和偏离标准的作战医疗保障原则方面的主要关切与数据缺失。其中最主要的是越来越多地使用规模更小、装备更差的队伍来提供高级外科治疗，并在支持作战行动时承担传统上任务 2 的全部或部分（如陆军高级外科团队）内容。这些团队现有各种规模和配置，一般不到 10 人，现被广泛称为"简朴的外科团队"。他们在完成部署前团队培训的数量和深度、设备和供应链，以及所支持的行动类型上也迥然不同。使用这些团队的最大问题之一是几乎完全缺乏客观数据来评估其有效性、优势和局限性以及患者结果。我们认为，与这些团队相关的改进的强制性数据收集分析最为重要，并应谨慎小心地使用这些数据，以确保实现可接受的护理和效果。除确定有关这些团队的研究重点外，目前外科战伤救治委员会（CoSCCC）还在制定一项新的联合创伤系统（JTS）临床实践指南，重点关注"简朴的外科团队"。

在"十大"研发重点中，人员和人员配置领域的其他研究重点与下列内容有关：确定任务 2 和任务 3 团队的最佳规模、人数和人员结构以及它们与各种手术环境结果的关系。除使用"简朴的外科团队"外，标准任务 2 和任务 3 团队的部署存在着重大变化且不定易变，其人员和专业组合也存在变化。任务 2 和任务 3 团队常被分为两个或多个更小的单位，每个单位都作为一个独立配备医疗设施支持前方作战。任务 2 团队的人员配置原则也发生了重大变化，最近的变化是增加了急救医疗人员，减少了外科医生的数量。这些变化的最终结果（如果存在）尚未得到深入的研究，应该成为国防部的另一个研究重点。最后，需要研究并分析确定手术团队人员、专业、培训的最佳组合，以便在苛刻的作战环境中达到最佳结果。尽管如此，这一领域是能说明多方面问题的优秀例证，即所需的解决办法不仅仅是简单的医学研究或研究经费，还需要在人员配置和培训理论、采购和装备、医疗规划和布局、强大的信息采集和分析等方面做出投入和改变。

复苏与出血管理

本重点领域与出血战伤患者的管理复苏相关，将其确定为优先研究重点并不令人意外，不同的研究项目均发现出血是可预防性战死最为常见的原因，也可支持本观点。这一结论与战术战伤救治委员会（CoTCCC）和途中救护委员会（CoERCC）确定的优先重点存在明显重叠。尽管大多数死亡发生在院前，且早期出血控制的研究大多针对于院前环境，但是一些对住院死亡的分析强调，出血控制仍然是到达有医疗设施（MTF）的机构后可预防的死亡和发病的最常见原因之一。本领域通过使用快速和间隙驱动的研究项目能明显看到巨大进步，并且在出血控制技术设备、培训项目和复苏策略方面取得了重大进展。

这一重点领域急需研究的几项被确定为本次分析的重中之重。随着血液制品日益成为首选的创伤失血患者第一复苏液，迫切需要研究下列方法：优化使用于恶劣环境中的血液制品，延长储存时间并简化储存要求，尽量减少输血时可能出现的相关并发症和不良反应。除了标准血液制品外，人们对药物辅料（如氨甲环酸）和凝血因子浓缩制品的兴趣也在不断增加，它们可能是复苏和纠正凝血障碍更为有效且高效的选择。出血控制显然需要有效的非手术干预措施，对于躯干出血尤为如此，非手术干预措施起到桥梁连接的作用，有利于向手术室的运送。目前，对于将复苏性主动脉球囊阻断术（REBOA）作为这一适应症的可行选择，人们存有很大兴趣，尽管还需要更多的研究来阐明适应症、技术、所需培训和方法，以尽量减少长时间复苏性主动脉球囊阻断术（REBOA）引起的缺血—再灌注。最后，高级环境中先进的有创监测在可及性和可用性方面是有局限的，所以另一个任务是开发和测试新的无创血液动力学监测系统，以帮助在早期识别严重出血或早期休克的患者，并指导复苏。

手术干预

由于任务 2 或更高级别设施的明显特征是存在外科医生与能够实施主要手术干预的

外科团队，因此该重点领域排名优先也就不足为奇。手术干预有别于先前的分析，此前的分析侧重于与固定的医疗设施（MTF）外部环境相关的问题。这一领域也与其他已经确定的重点领域有所重叠，例如出血患者的复苏，以及提供有效手术干预的最佳人员配置和能力。手术干预领域的新研究工作不仅需要考虑与严重战伤手术相关的一般问题，还必须考虑到不同类型部署部队的手术能力与主要任务的广泛差异。例如，部署的任务2 设施的核心责任通常仅限于实施重大损伤控制手术，然后转移到下一护理梯队。这与标准任务 3 设施的责任形成对比，任务 3 设施具备更强大的能力和容纳量，能够开展更为权威的手术治疗与更为复杂的重建手术。

除已经列出的围绕人员配置与能力结构的研究重点外，还需要开发用于重大损伤控制手术的改进技术和辅料，这应该是重中之重。促进拓宽外科医生控制出血和胃肠道溢液能力的新设备或技术可能与改善预后相关，也与提高保存稀缺资源（如血液制品和手术室时间）的能力相关。主要血管损伤管理的新进展也被列为十大研究重点之一，因为这些损伤往往最具挑战性，且最有可能导致不良后果。这点尤为重要，因为应届毕业的外科住院医师所接触的开放性血管手术与血管创伤病例越来越少，导致他们在战场上对这些损伤的确切处理缺乏经验，且感到不适，这一问题十分普遍。用以实现快速控制出血、重建动脉血流、实施临时或最终重建手术（如分流术、支架术、无缝线吻合术等）的辅料将需要进一步的重点研发规划。

结论

本论文初步制定分析了研究缺口和研究重点并列表排序，用以告知与战场外科护理任务 2 和任务 3 相关的战斗伤亡护理研究。本文包括一份"十大"研究重点列表，所有研究重点都来自三个重点领域，即人员和人员配置、复苏和出血控制以及主要手术干预。尽管本研究所包含的回复来自各个研究领域的专家组，我们发现评分和排序过程存在极高的一致性以及评估者间相关性。要解决高级外科治疗的挑战，除与以上优先重点一致的纯科学研究外，还需要改变军事理论、训练、教育、后勤、人员、设施和组织结构，这些都是联合创伤系统（JTS）和国防部其他部门的优先重点。

第五章　伤口护理和疼痛缓解

课文 A　未来的伤口护理

伤口，尤其是慢性伤口，从临床、社会和经济角度来看都是一个重大挑战。最近对美国医疗保险受益人所做的一项回顾性分析发现，大约有 820 万人都接受过至少一种类型的伤口治疗，其中外科手术切口和糖尿病溃疡是最常见且治疗费用最为高昂的伤口。此项研究还发现，与伤口护理相关的医疗保险支出远远高于此前的公认水平；急慢性伤口治疗的预估费用在 281 亿美元至 968 亿美元之间。

截至 2024 年，伤口护理产品的年度市场预计将达到 150 亿美元至 220 亿美元，但即便如此，伤口护理的很多方面依然是几十年不变。现在，由临床医生和技术人员组成的若干团队正致力于新技术的研发，希望能够从根本上改革伤口护理，使其更智能、快速和高效。

创新且安全的治疗方法

宾夕法尼亚州立大学农业和生物工程教授杰弗里·凯奇马克（Jeffrey Catchmark）主要研究方向是开发天然生物材料，以减少世界对塑料的依赖。为了找到聚苯乙烯泡沫塑料的替代品，他将一种阴离子淀粉和一种阳离子壳聚糖（一种从贝类外骨骼中提取的糖）结合起来，制成一种稳定的不溶性泡沫敷料。

凯奇马克发明的这种材料引起了宾州卫生署下属弥尔顿·S. 好时医疗中心创伤、急性护理和重症护理外科主任斯科特·阿蒙（Scott Armen）的兴趣，他同时也是美国陆军预备役的一名上校军官。他看到了这种新材料在伤口护理方面的应用潜力。阿蒙和凯奇马克利用这种新材料研发了一种生物泡沫敷料，可置于创伤伤口内，起止血和固定的作用。

这种材料开始时更像是一种传统泡棉，可吸收血液和体液，膨胀变大后还可起到压迫伤口的作用。随着愈合的进展，这种材料会进一步转化成一种凝胶，通过锁住创面的水分来帮助伤口愈合。此外，该生物泡沫还有其他一些非常吸引人的特性：其成分可生物吸收，长期使用安全；壳聚糖能促进凝血，有助于止血；该材料柔韧性好且持久耐用，可模制以更贴合地置于伤口内部。"到目前为止没有其他任何产品能以这种方式做到所有这些。"凯奇马克说。

凯奇马克和阿蒙希望能生产出一种可以外带的盒装泡沫敷料，便于携带，方便急救人员和军队医务人员在战地环境中使用。

凯奇马克说："这种材料最终可能会成为一种通用的伤口护理材料，可应用于几乎所有类型的伤口：创伤伤口、外科手术伤口或日常伤口。"

"从战场上的士兵到医院里的病人，甚至到日常家庭护理，它有可能真正影响人们的生活。"

按需随选的智能化解决方案

在哈佛医学院休假期间，萨米尔·松库西尔（Sameer Sonkusale）发现，他遇到的医生和临床医生最关心的就是伤口护理问题。"我们一直在用那种老式的绷带治疗伤口，治疗效果并不理想。"塔夫茨大学电气和计算机工程学院教授松库西尔说。受此启发，松库西尔与来自哈佛大学和普渡大学的同仁合作，开始研发一种可实时监控伤口愈合情况并按需提供治疗的方法。

其研究结果就是一种处于原型阶段的智能绷带。研究人员将其用于提高糖尿病小鼠的创口愈合程度，结果证明有效，它可以主动监测不同的伤口生物指标，在干预极少或零干预情况下准确给药。松库西尔说，柔性电子技术的出现使得我们能够设计一种同样具有柔韧性、足够薄、可用作绷带的智能材料。这种原型绷带包含加热元件和热反应药物载体，能够根据嵌入的 pH 和温度传感器（用于跟踪感染和炎症）提供定制剂量的抗生素或止痛药。通过提供伤口愈合情况的实时数据，并在必要时给药，这样的智能绷带可以为患者和医生节省时间和金钱。

"当伤口出现感染、需要更为密集的治疗时，问题就来了。"松库西尔说："我们想做的就是试图通过这种绷带建立一个闭环系统，监控绷带上的传感器，然后按需进行给药。"

虽然目前这个特制的原型绷带安装了 pH 和温度传感器以及抗生素给药系统，但松库西尔设想该绷带未来有更广泛的应用前景。绷带中内嵌的传感器类型及其可提供的治疗水平可以因人而异，以监测不同的愈合指标、处理不同的创伤情况。

虽然还需要进一步的临床试验以证明其有效性，但松库西尔认为智能绷带未来还有很大的进步空间，发展前景向好。

"我们做了几个版本的绷带，嵌入了一些特殊元件，以证明我们可以做到。"他说："但作为一个智能平台，我们的绷带将广泛适用于任何类型的伤口，包括烧伤、感染和糖尿病溃疡创面。"

以数据为驱动的远程管理

慢性创面和无法愈合的创面，如糖尿病溃疡，困扰着数百万美国人。最近的一项研究表明，近 15%的医疗保险受益人有至少一种慢性创面或感染需要治疗。为了满足这一需求，来自内布拉斯加州大学林肯分校、哈佛医学院和麻省理工学院的研究人员组成的一个团队设计了一种智能绷带，可以为这些不宜治愈的创伤口提供精准的、有针对性的药物治疗。

"这种绷带实现了两个方面的提升。"该绷带的发明者之一、康涅狄格大学生物医学工程系副教授阿里·塔马约尔（Ali Tamayol）说："一是给药方式，二是给药精度。"这种智能绷带配备有微型针头，能够深入伤口深层进行皮内给药，将患者的痛苦和炎症反应降到最低。这些针头均为无线控制，护理人员可以通过远程操作，制定合理的治疗方案并予以实施。

在用糖尿病小鼠进行的一项试点研究中，经过智能绷带治疗后，小鼠的创面显示出完全愈合和没有疤痕形成的迹象。与局部用药相比，该方法提高了伤口愈合的速度和质量。

塔马约尔说，他和他的合作者们都很重视听取护理人员和患者的意见，以此判断改进的方向。患者最关心的问题是尽量减少反复就医的频次，而护理人员更关心哪些措施可以让他们随时了解创面周围的环境情况。塔马约尔相信，这种智能绷带可以同时解决这两方面的问题。

塔马约尔说，可以通过更改智能绷带的一些组件，去适应不同类型伤口创面的需要。虽然智能绷带的应用前景和潜力让他激动不已，但他也承认，快速将这种产品推向市场依然要面临重重挑战。

"工程学领域的确出现了很多新兴、先进的技术，但将其应用于临床实践并不总是行得通的。"塔马约尔说："比较现实的操作可能是，在初期阶段先将其中一些技术简化后纳入临床实践，然后慢慢地再去加入一些更为复杂的技术。"

利用自然的生理运动

威斯康星大学麦迪逊分校材料科学与工程系教授王旭东（音译）十多年来一直致力于通过人体自身运动产生电能的研究，他开发了多种可穿戴设备，可将肌肉拉伸等身体运动转化为电能。他最近关注的研究方向是电脉冲对生物学过程的影响，尤其关注在医学上的应用。

"对于皮肤创面来说，实际上利用创伤部位的内部电场可以有助于细胞增殖。"王教授说："这就是为什么我们提出这个假设，即我们可以利用我们身体产生的电能来刺激伤口愈合，促进恢复。"

王教授和他的同事研发了一种绷带，通过利用身体自身的能量来加速愈合。这种绷带利用人体自身的运动在受伤部位产生温和的电脉冲，促进伤口愈合。该设备自带纳米发电机，可将诸如呼吸引起的人体运动转化为电脉冲。用一条绑带缠绕住患者（或实验动物）的躯干，并连接纳米发电机。患者（或实验动物）呼吸过程中胸腔的扩张和收缩会产生能量，可以带动纳米发电机，后者随之产生低强度的电脉冲，输入受伤部位。

在实验室试验中，用这种电子绷带治疗的大鼠在三天内伤口就完全愈合，而正常的愈合过程为两周。实验结果是令人鼓舞的，但王教授说，在这项技术进入人体试验之前，还需要做进一步的测试。他目前正在与威斯康星大学创伤和烧伤外科医生安吉拉·吉布森（Angela Gibson）合作，将这种电子绷带放在猪的身上进行测试（因为猪的皮肤与人类皮肤更为相似），同时他们也在实验室进行人类皮肤细胞的测试研究。

"我们已经在急性伤口上进行了试验，这可以让我们更好地研究细胞是如何反应的，但最终我们希望将这种技术应用于更为严重和更具挑战性的创伤上，如慢性创面和烧伤创面。"王教授说："烧伤创面覆盖面积大，且往往会留下疤痕。电场是有方向性的，这有助于细胞排列，从而尽可能地减少疤痕的形成。"

王教授相信，这项便捷高效、物美价廉的新型技术，除了用于伤口护理外，还可以有许多不同的治疗用途。他还研究论证了如何利用纳米发电机刺激毛囊生长，促进生发，以及如何利用纳米发电机刺激胃附近的迷走神经，使人产生饱腹感，以此来限制食物摄入和控制肥胖。

第六章　三防医学救治

课文 A　化学品伤亡管理基本事宜

本文概述了参与化学武器事故管理的医务人员应考虑的基本事宜。为有效管理此类事件，尤其是那些涉及大规模人员伤亡、因伤亡人数过多导致接诊人数骤增并超出医疗保障机构正常接待能力的化学品事故，必须对相关人员进行规划与培训。

应对化学武器事故要面临以下重要挑战：

1）化学试剂快速检测与鉴定。

2）风险规避，包括提供足够的防护和消毒，以及在受污染区域设置警戒线、实施出入管控。

3）伤亡人员消毒，不仅可减少受害人接触的化学试剂，同时也可避免污染扩散至医疗设施。

4）分诊和快速医疗处理，包括在事故现场和医院使用特效解毒剂进行治疗，以降低发病率和病死率。必须指出的是，医务人员可能要处理大批量的伤员，其中一些人甚至可能并没有中毒，而只是出现了心理症状。

化学品事故的管理是一个持续不断的过程，旨在减少或避免潜在的二次损害，确保向受害者提供及时且适当的援助，帮助他们迅速、有效地恢复。灾难管理基本周期包括以下几个阶段：

1）预防和减缓阶段：在事故发生前采取措施，通过评估危害和弱点，防止或尽量减少灾害影响。

2）准备阶段：基于第一阶段的评估，制定化学品事故管理计划，包括如何获取各种能力和人员培训方案。该管理计划应清楚明确地将地方、地区和国家各级医疗能力进行整合。可能需要制定相应的合作协议，协调不同服务和政府机构的能力，以便它们能够顺利纳入指挥和控制系统。事故管理计划应尽可能措辞简洁、表意清晰，因为复杂的计划往往难以实施。

3）响应阶段：实时事件发生时应急方案即时启动并付诸实施。响应阶段是否顺利取决于准备是否充分。

4）恢复阶段：最后阶段是采取相应措施使一切恢复到事故前的状态，包括处理危险材料、修葺事故现场，以及为受害者提供进一步的援助。

虽然上述四个阶段往往有部分重叠，且各阶段持续时间也会根据事故性质和严重程度而有所变化，但无论在哪个阶段，医疗管理都非常重要。

1. 检测（诊断）

化学武器事故发生之初，除非情报或执法部门事先发出警告，否则一线应急响应人员和医务人员不可能知道化学试剂的身份信息。此外，实验室对环境和临床样本进行鉴定后得到的准确的鉴定结果也需要时间才能反馈到医务人员手中。

目前可用于对化学武器中的化学试剂进行现场快速检测和鉴定的技术有很多种，包括（但不限于）：

离子迁移光谱法；

火焰光度法；

比色法/酶法；

表面声波器件；

光化电离；

傅里叶变换红外光谱法；

拉曼光谱法；

气相色谱法/质谱分析法。

所有便携式检测/鉴定设备，无论采用何种技术，受其灵敏度和选择的影响，都有可能会出现假阳性和假阴性的结果。如果只使用一种技术进行检测，那么这种检测可以说是"临时性的"，而如果使用至少两种不同技术进行检测，尤其是色度法或气相色谱/质谱法是其中之一时，则该检测的确信度水平更高。

虽然大多数便携式检测设备可以检测神经和糜烂性毒剂，但并不是所有设备都有能力检测其他的化学武器试剂。此外，这些设备大多是针对军事场景而设计，虽然一些应急单位可能配备了此类设备，但在民用场景中这些检测设备有可能会给出虚假反应。

由于所有这些原因，包括在某些情况下缺少可用的检测设备以及设备的敏感性和特异性不足，我们很有可能最早要通过中毒病人的体征和症状信息等迹象来判断是否使用了化学武器。

因此，医务人员应熟悉明确临床诊断、启动分诊程序所必需的主要体征和症状，为相关人员优先安排洗消和医疗救治。值得注意的是，这些临床表现的性质和出现时机不仅会随着暴露的持续时间和浓度而变化，而且也会随着暴露的途径而变化，在临床鉴别诊断和分诊过程中应予以考虑。例如，吸入的神经毒剂和氰化物（血液毒剂）起效快，需要立即治疗。

临床鉴别诊断还应考虑化学品接触带来的间接影响，包括穿戴防护装备引起的热应激、心理影响，甚至解毒剂的副作用，特别是在没有接触化学试剂但服用了解毒剂的情况下（例如，带有神经毒剂中毒解毒剂的自动注射器）。对于既有常规伤又有化学伤的混合伤，鉴别诊断和分诊可能会更为复杂。

2. 保护措施

化学攻击造成大规模人员伤亡事故中，医务人员是非常重要的资源。和其他事故响应人员一样，医务人员也是重要的保护对象，不能让他们成为受害者。个人防护装备（PPE）是化学污染环境中的第一道防线。个人防护装备包括防毒面具和防护服，包括大小适宜的手套和靴子。防毒面具尤其重要，因为化学品武器试剂通常是通过呼吸系统最大限度、最迅速地发挥作用。

通常情况下，中毒患者从污染区域转移出来并完成消毒程序之后，才会由医务人员接手进行后续治疗。但是，进入直接污染地区的一些应急服务机构的一线响应人员（例如，消防人员和执法人员）可以指派医务人员随行，以便为其行动提供医疗支持，进行早期医疗评估。在这些情况下，个人防护装备（PPE）可以保护医务人员，使其在直接接触受害者的皮肤、黏膜和衣服或在持续有毒气体环境中（特别是在狭小密闭空间里）呼吸时不会接触到化学试剂，防止其受到污染。

由于使用个人防护装备时，使用者的可视范围、机动性、灵活性和沟通能力都会受损，因此医疗管理的难度增加。此外，使用个人防护装备会加快新陈代谢、增加热产生、阻碍人体散热，从而增加热应激风险。在高温、高湿度和低风速等不利环境条件下，人体大量出汗导致快速脱水，会进一步恶化这种风险。因此，如果遇到有此类装备使用需要的灾害事故，参与人员必须身体健康并接受过个人防护装备适应性培训。

不同国家的个人防护装备和个人防护装备水平分类标准有所不同。最常用的分类标准，包括在禁止化学武器组织（OPCW）的援助和防护训练课程中使用的是美国环境保护署（EPA）的四级分类（参见表6-1）。各级防护水平主要体现在呼吸和皮肤防护上有所不同，通常根据化学试剂类型、毒性和浓度来选择不同的防护水平。

化学试剂身份特性未知、存在高浓度有毒试剂吸入风险、存在严重皮肤或黏膜损伤风险的情况下，应使用 EPA 分类中的 A 级防护用品，包括一套完全密封的、不透气的、耐化学腐蚀的防化服，耐化学腐蚀的内外层手套、鞋子或靴子，以及一个自给式呼吸器（SCBA）。如果发生泄漏，正压将允许空气从内部流向外部，但不会从外部流向内部。

需要最高级别的呼吸防护（包括缺氧环境）但对皮肤防护要求较低的情况下，使用 B 级防护用品。B 级防护必须包括自给式呼吸器（SCBA），但可以使用非密封防化服。

C 级与 B 级防护用品对皮肤防护的级别相同，但使用空气净化呼吸器（APR）代替了自给式呼吸器（SCBA）。目前市场上可以买到很多种不同类别和类型的过滤器，同时有一套既定的颜色编码系统，用以说明这些不同的过滤器可以过滤哪些化学物质。

D 级防护指普通工作服。医务人员常用的外科口罩、手术服和手套也被视为 D 级防护。在有呼吸或皮肤类化学武器试剂危险的场所不得使用此类防护用品。

表 6-1   美国环保署（EPA）个人防护装备四级分类

防护水平	呼吸防护	皮肤防护	使用场景
A 级	压力需求式全面罩自给式呼吸器（SCBA）	➢ 全密封防化服 ➢ 耐化学腐蚀的内外层手套和靴子/鞋	➢ 化学试剂未知 ➢ 化学试剂已知，但暴露风险极大（如高浓度、有飞溅风险、有浸入风险）
B 级	压力需求式全面罩自给式呼吸器（SCBA）	➢ 非密封连帽防化服 ➢ 耐化学腐蚀的内外层手套和靴子/鞋	➢ 化学试剂已知，对呼吸系统防护要求极高（对皮肤防护要求较低） ➢ 空气中含氧量低于 19.5%
C 级	全面罩或半面罩空气净化呼吸器（APR）	➢ 非封装连帽防化服 ➢ 耐化学腐蚀的内外层手套和靴子/鞋	➢ 化学试剂已知，环境浓度已知，且空气净化呼吸器可有效过滤环境中该浓度的化学试剂 ➢ 与已知化学试剂发生皮肤接触无危害，不会发生明显的透皮吸收 ➢ 空气中含氧量为 19.5% 及以上
D 级	无	➢ 普通工作服	➢ 无任何已知风险

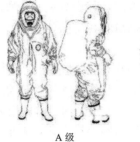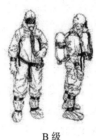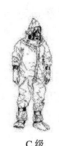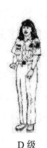

A 级　　　　　　　B 级　　　　　　C 级　　　　D 级

3. 医院管理

医院需要纳入灾害管理计划之中。只有这样，我们才能基于医院与受污染地区之间的距离，以及医院的接诊能力，妥善安排伤病员后送，并在救灾响应阶段不断调整更新，以维持患者的平衡分布。良好的沟通保障可以确保救护车数量充足，并在到达医院后驶入合适的接待区与医院对接。要将所有的医疗救治设施（机构）全部纳入灾害管理系统，这样一旦实验室通过检测最后得出了准确的鉴定结果，则能够确保该结果（即化学武器试剂的身份信息）可以全方位散播出去，从而确保为患者提供适当的医疗救治，包括对症的解毒疗法。

医院也应该有自己的应急预案。一旦启动，安保人员应控制人员和车辆进入医院，并引导他们进入接待区。受污染的患者有可能是自行到达，因此必须部署一条消毒走廊，通常在急诊科外或在一个预先划定好的区域。医院工作人员接触可能受污染的病人时应穿戴个人防护用品。通常 C 级防护足矣。

第七章　生物安全及应急响应

课文 A　医疗准备：以应对新冠病毒塑造医疗后勤的未来

去年 9 月新组建的陆军医疗后勤司令部（AMLC）启动时，我的重点很明确：准备我部在战略支援区（SSA）提供医疗物资和数据，以便在战术需要时达到支持作战部队的效果。我们知道我部即将在具有对抗性的多域环境中行动，因此我们需要迅速提高自身能力和承载力以实现上述效果。

组织变革从来都不是一件容易的事，尤其是我们正在进行系统性的作战医疗后勤改革。我们已预计到其时间漫长、道路崎岖且障碍重重。然而我们从未真正预料到的是一场全球性的大流行病。在我部发展不到 6 个月的时间里，我们发现自己处于陆军支持整个政府应对新型冠状病毒的中心位置。在整个夏季，陆军医疗后勤司令部（AMLC）持续为多个全球作战司令部提供医疗物资，以支持当前和未来的行动。

我们不曾预测到对新冠病毒的战斗，但它却为我们提供了独一无二的机会，来测试我们在具有对抗性的现实世界环境中，在战略支援区（SSA）达成效果的能力。

自 2018 年 10 月陆军医疗后勤部门开始建设以来，随着陆军医疗部门在国防卫生局（DHA）的领导下重新调整固定地点医疗服务的交付方式，我们见证了一段时期的重大变化，包括重组美国陆军医学研究和材料司令部（USAMRMC）与创建陆军医疗后勤司令部（AMLC）。

在长达 9 个月的时间里，陆军重组并停用了美国陆军医学研究和材料司令部（USAMRMC）。陆军总部的 013-19 号执行令要求立即将美国陆军医学研究和材料司令部（USAMRMC）移交给美国陆军器材司令部（AMC）。随后的 19-121 号作战令指示美国陆军医学研究和材料司令部（USAMRMC）"重组从而确保符合陆军未来部队的现代化要求"，并"制定一项详细的计划将医疗研发/项目管理移交给陆军未来司令部（AFC）"。到 2019 年 6 月 1 日，医学研究与物资部（MRMC）被重新指定为陆军未来司令部（AFC）下属的美国陆军医疗研究与发展司令部（MRDC）。

为了支持野战医疗后勤和部队，该命令还要求成立陆军医疗后勤司令部（AMLC），作为美国陆军器材司令部（AMC）的直属单位，于 2019 年 9 月 17 日启动。新的陆军医疗后勤司令部（AMLC）成为三个医疗后勤分司令部的总部：美国陆军医疗物资局、美国陆军驻韩医疗器材中心（USAMC-K）和美国陆军驻欧医疗器材中心（USAMC-E）。

创建陆军医疗后勤司令部（AMLC）属于几项更大的陆军医疗改革工作的一部分，这些改革旨在确保医疗准备就绪，支持战时需求，并提高士兵及其家属的护理质量。此外，陆军还力求将医疗后勤与陆军器材司令部（AMC）原有的其他维护职能集中起来。

陆军医疗后勤司令部（AMLC）为陆军提供医疗物资准备。我部与多个利益相关单位合作，确保医疗部队拥有所需的专业设备和物资，以便在战场内外继续为士兵提供最佳护理。我部通过综合医疗物资分配、前置库存、集中医疗物资管理和数据管理，为陆军作战部队和联合部队提供卫生服务保障，以支持大规模作战行动（LSCO）。

维持战略支援区行动

如今，陆军医疗后勤司令部（AMLC）是陆军的主要医疗后勤保障司令部，它提供对医疗物资的战略监督，涉及四大洲的陆军预置储备（APS）、前置库存、作战项目和医疗维持行动。我部在战略支援区（SSA）架构中支持陆军器材司令部（AMC）的四条工作线：

工业基地准备：

1. 为医疗设备和医疗专用测试、测量、诊断设备（TMDE-SP）提供保养维修、校准与资本重组。

2. 在作战环境部署医疗维修专家，提供高级维修与保养支持。

战略力量预测：

1. 管理维持医疗陆军预置储备（APS）、前置库存和其他医疗物资准备项目。

2. 提供前方作战的光学制品制造，包括标准版眼镜和自选框架眼镜，防毒面具和眼部防护的插入件，以及飞行员的飞行护目镜。

3. 与美国国务院合作协调医疗对外军售（FMS），加强盟国合作伙伴的实力，确保互通互用。

供应保障与设备准备：

1. 监督整个陆军和联合医疗部队的医疗物资（例如，补给、装备和装配）分发。

2. 分发疫苗并提供冷链管理培训。

3. 支持医疗物资质量控制与危险品召回。

4. 为陆军和联合医疗部队提供战区级医疗后勤保障。

数据分析与后勤信息准备：

1. 促进陆军医疗后勤从传统的企业资源规划（ERP）系统过渡到全球作战支援系统-陆军（GCSS-Army），最迟于2022财年底完成。

2. 管理并更新医疗物资目录。

3. 提供技术业务支持和记录系统培训。

与新冠病毒斗争

美国首例高传染性新型冠状病毒病例于1月21日确诊。3月11日，世界卫生组织（WHO）宣布其为全球大流行病，这对众多美国人而言是疫情战斗的开始。但在陆军医疗后勤司令部（AMLC），这场战斗早在几周前就开始了。

美国大陆以外的战区保障

医疗物资配送。随着美国国内的病例开始增多，陆军医疗后勤司令部（AMLC）收到命令，通过美国北方陆军（USARNORTH）作为美国陆军北方司令部（USNORTHCOM）的联合部队陆上分队指挥部，为地方当局提供防务支持（DSCA）。

到3月份，陆军医疗后勤司令部（AMLC）为纽约州和华盛顿州的三个陆军医院中心分发了医疗用品，这两个州最先遭到新冠病毒重创。这项任务包括从肯塔基州坎贝尔堡的531医院中心、科罗拉多州卡森堡的627医院、得克萨斯州胡德堡的第九医院中心向陆军医疗专业人员提供支持。其部队部署计划（UDP）包括根据每个医疗队的需要定制药效及有效期，包括注射器、吸管、血液制品和氧气等各种物资，旨在加强这些单位的能力，在最需要的地方提供卫生保健支持。

利用陆军预置储备。与此同时，陆军医疗后勤司令部（AMLC）继续在世界范围内为应对大流行病提供支持。在欧洲，我部从陆军预置储备中发放医疗物资，包括呼吸机、病人监护仪和病床，供德国兰施图尔（Landstuhl）区域医疗中心使用。我们还向包括美国中央总部（USCENTCOM）行动区的多个海外地点发放野战医院装备，以增强全球的陆军能力。我部在美国各地为美国陆军北方司令部（USNORTHCOM）预置了呼吸机和呼吸机补给包。

整合全陆军的支持机构。医疗后勤是精简的专业。为了完成任务，特别是在新冠疫情期间，陆军医疗必须与其他机构整合同步。建立我部并将我部作为陆军器材司令部（AMC）下属的主要司令部，其益处便在此时显现。在陆军装备司令部（AMC）内部，与其他直属单位和战友团队的整合同步有助于陆军医疗后勤司令部（AMLC）缓解在储存、人力和配送能力方面的不足与差距，同时为医疗维护任务提供独特的支持能力。

与合作伙伴和主要利益相关者合作。陆军很少单独部署，因此所有军事服务之间的协调以及与盟军合作伙伴的互通性至关重要。陆军医疗后勤司令部（AMLC）通常直接与下列单位合作：

1. 国防后勤局部队保障司令部（DLA-TS）负责管理战略医疗物资的获取、分配和准备计划。

2. 陆军未来司令部（AFC）和美国陆军医疗研究与发展司令部（USAMRDC）将后勤的生命周期管理职能与项目管理职能和活动结合起来，以开发和交付可持续的装备解决方案。

3. 国防卫生局（DHA）执行国防医疗后勤计划和共享服务，如物资标准化和数据管理。

4. 国防医疗后勤企业和美国陆军医疗司令部/美国公共卫生署署长办公室合办论坛和倡议行动，以促进装备标准化和联合操作互通性。

5. 陆军军种组成司令部（ASCCs）和作战司令部制定并执行医疗服务保障计划的医疗后勤部分。

6. 美国陆军部队司令部（FORSCOM）及其下属司令部负责医疗部队的现代化和准备工作、可安装级别的医疗供应、维修和光学制品制造。

在对抗新冠病毒的过程中，这些已经建立的关系变得尤为宝贵。从洗手液到检测试剂盒再到个人防护用品，多种资源很快就供不应求。我部加入了联合优先分配委员会，并与利益攸关方合作，精心安排基于需求的医疗物资交付。

重建能力。维持任何长期的战斗都需要前瞻性的思维策略，维持对抗新冠病毒的战斗也不例外。到目前为止，我部已经建立了强化流程来快速填补药效和过期物品，以及诸如呼吸机气管等耗材。这项持续性保障工作的关键部分之一便是与供应商和国防后勤局部队保障司令部（DLA-TS）的合约，这为我们提供了采购速度和灵活性。

我们还必须创造性地思考如何分配和维持物品供应。就传统意义而言，我们是流动的队伍。我们的模式要求实际前往一个部队或部署地点，将医疗后勤保障组（MLST）投放到库存和发放物品上。在对抗性环境中，新冠疫情的出行限制迫使我们改变行动计划。

我们在网上举办了虚拟培训研讨会，并为许多医疗设备制作了维护提示单，总结出解决这些问题最为关键的细节。我们直接与全球的医疗维护人员和单位共享这些产品。我们的网站也作为知识库保障医疗维护团体，提供建议表单和几十个常见问题。

我们实施了"远程维护"，将维修人员与现场单位虚拟地连接起来，以协助排除故障和维修复杂的医疗设备。尽管尚处于早期阶段，我们相信这一努力将为我们扩展资源，充分利用医疗维护运转部（MMODs）的原有专业知识带来巨大影响。

陆军医疗后勤司令部（AMLC）的未来之路

在统领发展的同时，我们在五个方面进行了重点改革，以应对挑战、弥合差距、开拓机遇。

可视与集成。作为商品，第八类（医疗）补给长期以来一直在努力实现首端到末端的可视性，并融入陆军的主要企业资源规划系统，即全球作战支援系统—陆军（GCSS-Army）。新冠疫情未能确认这一问题，它进一步突显了差距，以及我们无法审视自身的问题。好消息在于我们正在着手解决这个问题，而且开始将第八类（医疗）补给整合到全球作战支援系统—陆军当中。我们首先从陆军预置储备着手，这样一来它就可以像其他商品一样受到管理，并为部队领导提供更好的可视性。在美国陆军联合兵种支援司令部（CASCOM）和通信与电子司令部（CECOM）的共同领导下，我们将很快把全球作战支援系统—陆军的第八类（医疗）补给从战术层面重新整合到工业基地。这项工作将从 2020 财年第四季度开始，并于 2022 财年末完成，实现全面整合。

分配。陆军医疗后勤司令部（AMLC）负责作战医疗后勤，但是美国军事处理设施（MTFs）的医疗后勤仍隶属于国防卫生局（DHA）。尽管如此，我们必须共同努力，以避免采购内耗与效率低下。我们目前正在制定一个新修订的保障概念，更好地整合整个机构的第八类（医疗）物资配送，并确保对于需要从这些地点获取现有物资的部署部队，国防卫生局的治疗设施（DHA MTF）仍然是其备用供应源。

规划与响应。通过雇佣需求规划员、确定战备驱动因素、利用国防后勤局（DLA）的医疗应急需求工作流程，陆军医疗后勤司令部（AMLC）正在提高其需求规划能力，以便向国防后勤局的医疗应急档案提供更准确的信息，该档案确定了联合、分时段的"开战"医疗物资需求。我们的总体目标是尽早向工业基地发出准确的需求信号，以便工业基地在必要时能够激增产量满足需求。

管理与维护。陆军医疗后勤司令部（AMLC）未来将发展成为生命周期管理司令部（LCMC），配备物资经理、后勤援助代表、国家级采购部门和专家级高级司令部代表，能够在兵团和设施层面提供直接保障。我们必须与美国陆军医疗研究与发展司令部（USAMRDC）的项目经理和装备开发者合作，从初建到撤资或现代化，改进第八类（医疗）装备的管理和维护计划。

能力与承载力。或许我们从新冠疫情中学到的最重要一课是它挑战了我们先前所拥有的假设和思维过程。在传统上，陆军医疗后勤所计划的医疗物资需求针对于战场环境中军人最常见的战斗伤亡或疾病。我们可以理解，创伤所需的医疗物资（外科手术和血液）类型与大流行病所需的医疗物资（呼吸机和制氧设备）类型大不相同。它们的消耗率，或者说消耗物品的速度，也是不同的。在战斗护理环境中，只有医护人员佩戴个人防护装备。在流行病中，因为非医疗服务提供者也需要个人防护装备，其消耗率远高于之前。

新冠肺炎疫情教会了我们重新思考补给的一些计划因素。我们一直在与临床医生和药剂师密切合作，开发新的成套项目，以保障快速灵活地补充一次性部件，如呼吸机等医疗设备上的管线和阀门。这种思维的转变不仅有助于我们更好地保障应对当前的大流行病，而且还将影响我们如何维持未来的作战行动。

最后的思考

虽然陆军医疗后勤司令部（AMLC）的转变并非由新冠肺炎疫情引起，但我们从这场战斗保障中学到的东西极大地影响了我们的改革工作。在每一次挑战中，我们都努力寻找机会，更快、更有效地做好准备。在许多方面，保障新冠肺炎抗疫的任务使我部更好地了解了在多域环境（包括大规模作战行动）中如何满足大规模和指数级医疗物资的需求。

我部目前所处的对抗性环境是对未来的预演。作为一个超级体育迷，我经常向全世界的指挥官和参谋们解释如今的挑战："没有机会单手上篮。"战场上一切都强调输赢。在恰当的时间交付正确的工作，这一道路常常崎岖不平，我们必须积极进取——但是我们已经在前进的路上。

第八章　战斗行动压力控制

课文 A　深入剖析美军日益严重的心理与行为问题

值阿富汗及伊拉克战事方酣之际，首先要谈的是伤亡数——美军阵亡与负伤的惨烈记录，随之就是参战官兵患有创伤后应激障碍与创伤性脑损伤的问题。

美军正在苦于应对部队内部层出不穷的心理与行为问题——从药物成瘾、重度忧郁、自杀，乃至于虐待配偶与其他暴力行为、节节攀升的离婚率、犯罪、酗酒以及虐待孩童等。此境况如今已逐渐受到军队医疗人员、军方高层、退伍军人团体以及国会的重视。

2008 年 6 名原驻于科罗拉多州卡森堡的退伍军人被控在过去 12 个月内杀害 8 人。军方随即对这起疯狂射杀事件的原因展开调查，而该事件也使卡森堡一夕成名，更凸显了有效处理退伍军人日趋严重行为问题的必要性。2009 年 7 月发布的调查报告指出，暴露在战斗环境所造成的影响，是其行凶原因之一。

兰德公司的新研究报告估计，从阿富汗及伊拉克返国的 70 万名军人中，约有 18.5%检测出患有创伤后应激障碍或忧郁症，另有 19.5%已罹患轻重度创伤性脑损伤。

更惊人的数据来自旧金山退伍军人福利管理局医疗中心内科诊所的一份研究报告（2009 年 9 月刊载于《美国公共卫生月刊》）。该报告中指出，在伊拉克及阿富汗服役后进入退伍军人医疗体系的成员中，超过 1/3 的退伍军人已经诊断出心理健康问题。若加上心理社会及行为失调者，人数将提升 40%。

1. 与部署有关？

对许多美国人而言，不难看出导致此种问题的原因。从当下城市战斗与戡乱的情况看，战斗的紧凑程度不言而喻。况且有些部队是反复部署至战区2次、3次，甚至达到4次之多。

评论人士认为，这些由部署所产生的压力——无论是实际投入战斗的陆军官兵及陆战队员，还是置身于战区外的支援人员，为使作战行动得以顺利进行，均须格外努力且经常超时工作，这已经对官兵的身心造成伤害。而目前的"轮休期"——部队再次部署前得以返国的时间——不超过1年而已。

曾任美空军军医主任，并担任国防部有关战区服役官兵医疗问题顾问的退役空军中将罗德曼二世表示："大家讨论的是一支兵疲马困的部队。这种形态的战争较我们以往认知中的战争更具压迫感，实际上官兵时刻都在战斗。"

2. 高优先性

美军心理卫生的问题现已到了军方及地方领导公开承认，并亟须着手处理的地步。国防部长盖茨表示："除了打赢战争外，我最优先的工作就是为作战官兵提供最佳的医疗服务，包括那些饱受心理及行为问题折磨的人员。"

各军种均表示已开始筛检更多从阿富汗及伊拉克返国的部队。4个军种部都制定了可尽早发现与治疗心理及行为问题的计划，并成立"官兵调适"单位以治疗并支持负伤官兵。

各军种也倾向准许部队在两次部署之间能有较长的"轮休时间"，使其可利用再度回到战区前，能更充分地适应国内生活，纾解紧张的战斗压力。在某些状况下，陆军或陆战队官兵轮休不过数月再度回到战区，心理学家认为，这么短的时间对官兵得到良好适应来说是远远不够的。

国防部成立了6所"心理健康与创伤性脑损伤国防卓越中心"，结合军方、退伍军人管理单位及地方力量共同研究和治疗心理疾病，此举措极具深远影响。美陆军近期斥资5000万美元针对自杀及心理卫生问题展开研究，以期探究当前问题的原因及治疗方法。

3. 心理卫生人员短缺

面对官兵日益增加的心理疾病，一个主要的难题就是各军种尚缺受过训练的心理卫生人员。马里兰大学的席格教授指出，尽管国防部在这两场战争开战之初，迅速向战区部署了医疗人员，然而由于没有考虑两场战事的持续时间与参战部队人数，导致医疗人员的部署人数远远不够。

国防部心理卫生小组在2007年做出的结论指出：目前心理卫生专业人员的数量严重不足。而众议院在2008年所提法案中也指出，陆军需要合格临床心理医师的空缺职位约有40%，其他包括精神病治疗与临床社会工作在内的心理卫生专业人员也不足。

此外，位于纽约的退伍军人团体——美国驻伊拉克及阿富汗退伍军人协会表示，驻伊拉克美军得到的心理卫生保障实际上正在减少。2004年，该战区平均每387名美军仅有1名行为保健工作者，2007年该比例降为每734名美军只有1名。陆军或陆战队官兵转诊至精神科医生或心理专家所需时间也大大超出了正常规定时间。

各军种始终致力扩充其医疗人力资源，但迄今某些类别的医疗人员数量仍显不足。美国国防部的数据显示，2008 年美军共有 308 名现役精神科医生，较核定数少 4.5%；另有 584 名心理专家，较核定数少约 14%，况且核定人数并未反映实际需求数量。

退伍军人共识协会和驻伊拉克及阿富汗退伍军人协会两个团体都积极向国会提出增加精神卫生专家的要求，并要求部队官兵在派驻战区前和返国后，强制进行面对面的心理测验。

4. 治疗不断改进

因果关系的不确定性并不代表各军种对治疗心理及行为问题束手无策。即便是最苛刻的批评者也承认，军方在治疗这类病情上已有显著进步。许多人认为，军方是鉴别和治疗这些疾病的佼佼者，而近来军方更被认为是治疗这类疾病的开拓者，因为这类疾病在地方医疗机构看来也同样是棘手的问题。

美国国防医科大学精神病学系主任厄撒诺博士表示，未来数月军队医疗将面临的主要工作之一，就是审查近年来成立的精神卫生方案，移除那些功能重叠或效果不佳的项目，再扩大一些效果明显的方案。他说："此项工作属于修正性质，一旦数据获得无误，就会将建议反馈军方，以利于这项工作的具体落实。"

这些工作才刚刚起步。国防卓越中心的苏藤将军指出："我们此刻的挑战就是要在医疗界全面推行该工作，使其尽可能加速进行。拖得越久对我们越不利。"

第九章　精准医疗

课文 A　精准医疗：仍然存在哪些障碍？

精准医疗在推动更有针对性的治疗和更健康的社会方面，前景一片光明。但事实证明，个性化医疗的实施并不顺利，那么还存在哪些问题阻碍了其充分发挥潜力呢？

自古以来，个体的重要性就在医学界得到了广泛认可。自 19 世纪以来就有了医生应该"治疗病人，而不是治疗疾病"这句广为流传的格言，而人们对此的认识还要远远早于这一时间。在公元前 5 世纪行医治病的"西方医学之父"希波克拉底，就强调将每个病人作为个体来治疗的重要性。

希波克拉底写道："甜[药]不能使每个人都受益，苦药不能使每个人都受益，也不是所有的病人都能喝同样的药剂。"

希波克拉底可能是根据病人的年龄、体质和其他容易观察到的因素来调整基本治疗方法，到了 21 世纪，个性化医疗则有望实现定制治疗，其研究依据正是使我们真正具备独一无二属性的 DNA。

个性化医疗的前景

基因组学、蛋白质组学、数据分析和其他医学和技术领域的进步正在不断促进精准药物的开发，使我们得以预测个体罹患特定疾病的风险因素以及个体对各种治疗可能有何不同反应。

经过多年期盼，现在有证据表明，世界各国政府已经认识到个性化医疗的重要性，并且正在推进建立基因数据集和生物库的工作，而这正是推动科学发展所需要的。2015年，美国前总统巴拉克·奥巴马大张旗鼓地发起了"精准医疗计划"，该计划后来演变成为"全民健康研究计划"，旨在收集超过一百万美国志愿的健康数据，以获得新的发现。

在英国，"十万个基因组计划"已实现目标，完成了对免费医疗体系中 8.5 万名癌症或罕见疾病患者的 10 万个全基因组的测序工作。英格兰基因组学协会指出，到目前为止，对这些数据的分析已在大约四分之一的罕见疾病患者身上发现了"可操作的研究结果"，大约 50%的癌症病例也表明有可能进行治疗或临床试验。

"输血时匹配血型——这是一个重要的发现。"奥巴马在"精准医疗计划"的启动仪式上说，他总结了个性化治疗和诊断的广泛用途。"如果癌症治疗与我们的遗传密码匹配也能如此简单，如此标准呢？如果确定准确的药物剂量就像测量体温一样简单呢？"

早期：临床应用进展缓慢

个性化医疗的舞台可能已经搭好，将极大地改变公共卫生，但在医学领域很少有人会否认这个世界还没有准备好。从传统的一刀切治疗模式过渡到利用患者的基因、生活方式和环境风险因素的新模式是一项艰巨的任务，给实验室和临床都带来了挑战。

肿瘤学绝对是受精准医疗发展影响最大的领域。2018 年批准上市的顶级精准治疗中，约 90%是癌症治疗，其他治疗领域则远远落后。大多数获批的肿瘤学精准治疗都在新旧方法之间实现了某种程度的折中——虽然没有达到为特定个体量身定做的程度，但已经能够根据患者肿瘤的致癌突变（这些突变可能推动了癌细胞的存活和生长）对患者进行更详细的分层。

常见突变包括某些乳腺癌和胃癌中的 HER-2、黑色素瘤中的 BRAF 和肺癌中的 EGFR。这些蛋白质在癌症部位的高表达可以通过精准治疗来靶向，如罗氏针对 HER-2 的单克隆抗体赫赛汀（曲妥珠单抗）、基因泰克的 BRAF 抑制剂 Zelboraf（威罗非尼），以及罗氏的 EGFR 抑制剂 Tagrisso（奥西替尼）。美国食品药品监督管理局和欧洲药品管理局等监管机构还批准了更多"肿瘤位置未知"疗法，其中第一个也是最著名的是默克公司的免疫疗法 Keytruda（派姆单抗）。该疗法靶向的是特定生物标记物，而不考虑肿瘤位于何处。

然而，尽管个性化癌症治疗方案越来越多，实际上为患者找到合适的治疗方法可能却很困难。权威医疗（Definitive Healthcare）开展了一项针对美国急性护理组织的调查，根据 2019 年 12 月发布的调查结果，仅有约 20%的机构制定了精准医疗计划。对基因组检测的投资对于迅速让患者接受最佳治疗方案至关重要，但资金和操作障碍依然存在。

其中最重要的是与基因组测序和配套诊断设备相关的成本，在权威医疗（Definitive Healthcare）的调查中，28%的受访者认为这是现有精准医疗计划面临的最大挑战。缺乏专业知识是另一个障碍，因为许多医生可能难以在没有专家协助的情况下准确解释检测结果。这是诊所和医院想要打造掌握最新检测技术的病理团队的另一个主要成本驱动因素。2018 年卡地纳健康（Cardinal Health）对 160 名肿瘤医生的调查发现，未使用基因组检测的医生中有 60%是因为难以解释数据而避免使用此类检测。

精准医学在药物开发领域面临的障碍

在临床研究和开发领域，将药研发管线转向针对小规模患者亚群也面临越来越多的烦恼。同样，成本也是一个核心问题——辅助诊断并不便宜，寻找和验证生物标记物以指导靶向治疗也是一项漫长的任务，而分析大量数据通常还需要具有专业知识的新团队。

将大量新流程纳入创新试验设计的费用，更不用说制造细胞和基因疗法的成本，显然会对获得批准的个性化药物的标价产生影响。这一点在世界上第一批真正的个体化癌症治疗——嵌合抗原受体 T 细胞（CAR-T）疗法——令人瞠目的价格中体现得淋漓尽致。

诺华公司的 Kymriah 和吉利德公司的 Yescarta 等疗法从病人血液中取出 T 细胞，将其进行改造成靶向肿瘤细胞抗原，然后输回血液中。这些疗法在罕见癌症和晚期癌症中取得了令人瞩目的效果，但每位患者的费用超过 40 万美元，限制了私人和公共支付方的报销选择。在 CAR-T 制造和潜在的"现成的"T 细胞生产方面，大有希望的进展可能有助于在未来几年降低这些成本，但目前费用问题仍然存在。

至于更广泛的临床试验生态系统，这些研究历来都用于评估候选药物在越来越多的患者群体中的安全性和有效性，为监管部门审批提供证据。在临床开发过程中引入个性化医疗在许多方面都是一种新的范式。除了上述成本驱动因素外，确定和招募患者还可能产生额外负担，这本就是试验失败的一个常见原因，但如果希望寻找的是具有适当生物特征的小规模患者亚群，就会更加困难。

监管的不确定性

难以提供充分的安全性和有效性证据也可能导致当前的法规很难应对个性化医疗的创新范式。小型试验设计在理解药物的明确风险－收益方面会存在统计学问题。此外，在一些大型临床试验中可以发现某些"个性化"应用，但除了具有某些生物标记物的特定人群，这些大型试验并未在整个研究人群中达到预计的终点。当前的许多法规并不接受这种事后分析，还要求开展一个完整的新的临床试验。

"个性化医疗开发者希望得到更好的指导，了解如何以最佳方式设计成功的个性化疗法临床试验，因为如果没有指导，他们在分层选择时就有可能提供次优证据。"2017年发表在《法律与生物科学杂志》的一项关于个性化医疗障碍的研究指出："为不同反应亚组（例如，生物标记物阳性组和生物标记物阴性组）设计临床试验需要额外的时间和资源，在获得监管部门批准的确定性没有相应提高的情况下，企业就不愿进行这种投资。"

更多替代终点、有条件批准和真实世界数据的使用有助于解决这些问题，但它们还不是理想的解决方案。有条件批准依赖于非常详细的上市后观察和分析，而替代终点的价值一直受到质疑，加剧了加速批准和确保患者安全之间的矛盾。

研发更多个性化治疗的终极收益显而易见，从长远来看，它们的经济回报会与其对人类健康的益处相匹配。毕竟，对负担过重的卫生系统来说，用适合患者的疗法快速开展治疗——或者更好的是，利用遗传风险信息事先预防疾病——将带来巨大的经济收益。

正如美国国立卫生研究院有关 DNA 测序成本的数据所示，如今的成本正在逐渐下降。但是，即使在领先的肿瘤学领域，想要告别几十年来主导现代制药的全方位药物开发，还有很长的路要走，更不用说其他治疗领域了。只有来自监管机构、药物开发人员、临床医生、政府和其他方面持续和全面的努力，才足以推动我们跨过药物研发这条界限。

第十章　智慧军事医疗

课文 A　为什么超级战士可能很快噩梦成真

早在 1941 年 3 月美国队长就首次与观众见面，随后在漫威电影《美国队长：复仇者先锋》中，瘦骨嶙峋的孩子一跃成为强壮彪悍的英雄，超级战士这个概念也因而从 40 年代进入现代人意识当中。从那时起，就不乏有文章将美国队长这位英雄与正在进行的提升人类最大潜能的研究进行对比，但这些工作究竟有多少实际意义呢？事实证明，它们越来越有可能成为现实。

当然，很重要的一点是要记住，并不是每一项提升人类表现的科学研究本质上都与军事有关。虽然美国队长在达到人类能力巅峰的过程中受益于国防研究，但如今私营制药集团和大学支持的研究人员在提高人类表现方面也取得了重大进展。在真正打造全方位 "超级战士" 的工作中，几乎可以肯定私营部门的研究、治疗，甚至身体改造工程会发挥重要作用，确切地说，这可能还是五角大楼更青睐的模式。

近年来，国防部越来越重视利用私营部门已经开发的 "现成" 技术。与传统的征求建议和签订研发合同等方式相比，利用 "现成" 技术能够节省大量成本，并且大大加快交付速度。一个新的国防项目利用的现成组件越多，它从理论变成现实的速度就越快。这一思路不仅适用于研发步枪和夜视镜，还可能适用于五角大楼希望成功部署超级士兵所需的医疗和技术。

因此，让我们来了解一些国防和私营部门的项目，它们可能确实有助于推动战场上超级英雄时代的到来。

工程化血液可以大幅提升性能

人体是为一种相当严格的生活方式而设计的，但在不太遥远的将来工程设计的人造红细胞可能真正使未来的超级士兵具备比竞争对手更多的优势。这些人造红细胞被称为呼吸细胞，可以让使用者长时间屏住呼吸，并大幅提升心血管耐力。

这些微型机器只由三部分组成：吸收和释放氧气的转子、吸收和释放二氧化碳的转子，以及吸收和释放葡萄糖的转子。实际上，呼吸细胞的功能和红细胞一样，但性能远远优于大自然的设计。这个概念基于分子制造研究所纳米技术研究员罗伯特·弗雷塔斯的工作，能够让使用者 "在游泳池底部屏住呼吸四小时，或全速冲刺至少 15 分钟而不用停下来呼吸"。

能够屏住呼吸数小时显然对于海上登陆的特种作战人员很有帮助，而且这些超级细胞提供的额外耐力在地球上几乎所有战斗环境中都会派上用场。

夜视功能可以直接注射进眼睛

如今，战场上美军经常使用夜视镜，但这些夜视镜确实存在一些缺陷。配发给地面部队的标准夜视镜提供的周边视野很少，深度感知更差，难以适应危险行动，而且增加了危险行动的风险，比如高速驾驶或与敌人交火。特种作战部队通常配有更好的夜视装备，最近民用夜视镜上市，但每副价格 4 万美元左右。这些功能更强大的夜视镜成本过高，无法大规模配发部队……但如果我们不再需要它们呢？

马萨诸塞州伍斯特市马萨诸塞大学医学院最近的一项研究中，小鼠被训练沿着一路上遇到的三角形标志在迷宫中行走。随后，在关灯的情况下，研究人员让小鼠再次尝试，结果和预期一样：它们在黑暗中找不到路。然后，科学家向小鼠的眼球中直接注射了能将红外光转换为可见光的纳米粒子，结果是小鼠获得了新的视觉能力，能够在黑暗中视物，这种能力可以持续约 10 周，而且似乎没有任何副作用。

在战场上将意念转化为战斗力

尽管美国队长拥有多项技能，他却从未成功掌握读心术或心灵感应，但未来这些技能可能会成为标配。十年前，美国国防部高级研究计划局已经在试验能够实现"无声交谈"的头盔。其目的是在使用者说话前读取他的脑电波，并将其转换为可传输的数据。随后接收者的系统接收这些数据并将其转换成听觉或视觉信号。

这将使战场上的士兵能够在保持完全静默的情况下进行交流，但这种技术的用途远不止与班长悄声密语。2018 年，美国国防部高级研究计划局宣布，一名装有实验脑机接口的人，成功地用意念同时控制了三种不同类型的模拟飞机。

这一技术可以让战斗机飞行员通过意念无缝地控制空军的"天空星"或波音公司的"忠诚僚机"等项目中配备了人工智能的无人机僚机。在未来，同样的技术还可以用于其他无人机和半自动地海空平台——允许战斗人员携带自己的重型增援装备，甚至控制他们穿戴的机器人外骨骼参加战斗。

像美国队长一样使用药物

美国队长注射超级战士血清最重要的功能是把他从一个瘦小羸弱的身躯变成一个重量级冠军，但这是否真的可行？

类固醇和其他提高性能的药物已经存在一段时间，毫无疑问，已经有这类药物被用于军事用途的先例。然而，使用合成代谢类固醇需要配备精心控制的治疗计划，包括利用药物抵消身体产生更高水平的雌激素，从而抵消身体系统中增加的睾酮。如果不能有效管理荷尔蒙就会导致严重的健康问题，包括我们从小到大听到的健美运动员注射药物的各种情况。

根据维多利亚大学生物医学研究中心主任 E. 保罗·泽尔的说法，已经用于治疗、治愈病人或为其提供补充的激素和基因疗法最终可以用于将普通士兵变身为超级战士。

泽尔认为，类似的治疗方法可以用来将一个人的身体能力推进到人类潜能的极限。他引用了家畜研究的一些做法，比如从比利时蓝牛身上去除肌肉生长抑制素基因，让它们长出大量的肌肉，称其真实展示了人类受试者的未来可能性。他认为，将这些治疗方法与临床开发的训练方案结合起来，可能让普通人比连队里最强健的健身达人还要强壮30%。

目前几乎可以肯定的是，未来的战场上将会出现这样或那样的超级战士——无论他们是基因、生物还是技术改造的产物（或者可能三者兼有）。一马当先并不总是意味着性能最佳，就像之前的军备竞赛一样，在这个过程中肯定会有一些惊喜。